What Reviewers and Readers have to say about...
How to Teach Nutrition to Kids

"...an excellent resource for those in the position of teaching nutrition to children..."
— *Journal of the American Dietetic Association*

"...one of the most creative books you'll find on nutrition or on activities in any of the discipline areas. Outstanding."
— *Teaching K-8, The Professional Ideabook for Teachers*

"Evers does a fantastic job integrating fun with healthy choices...students will learn essential information that should keep them thinking — and eating — healthy for years to come."
— *Teacher's Edition Online*

"Wow!...a wonderful tool for all educators who work with children. The book is divided into sections that make it very easy for teachers to implement nutrition with other subjects. Yet the numerous activities will have children improving their eating habits from day one! Ms. Evers has clearly written this for today's children and the many pitfalls they have in their diet and lifestyle. *How to Teach Nutrition to Kids* is fun and educational for all ages and is a valuable teacher's tool."
— *The Science Spiders™ Newsletter*

"Provides a vast supply of practical hands-on activity ideas. These ideas are creative, fun-focused and easy to put into action."
— *VENTURES Newsletter*

"Parents, as well as teachers, will find a lot of fun, hands-on activities in this book."
— *The Oregonian*

"Evers' philosophy is to keep nutrition education child-centered. In her book she offers dozens of activities for both teachers and parents to empower kids to make good choices."
— *The Chicago Tribune*

"Evers writes well, employing a brisk style that makes everything clear without being simplistic. This book holds out the opportunity for parents and schools to cooperate in helping children develop healthy eating and exercise habits."
— *The Statesman Journal (Salem, OR)*

"This up-to-date, easy-to-read book and guide are packed with creative activities that will appeal to children and make their learning more fun and meaningful. The book and leader/activity guide would be valuable resources for anyone interested in teaching kids about good nutrition."
— *Wellness Web*

"...delightful and so helpful, just filled with great, usable ideas... a great contribution to those of us that teach."
— *Iowa youth nutrition leader*

"...your writing is wonderful; and I've certainly promoted your book to health educators in our state..."
— *Missouri dietitian*

"I would like to compliment you on your book. I've been recommending it to everyone!"
- *State Nutrition Education & Training Coordinator*

24 Carrot Press
P.O. Box 23546
Portland, OR 97281-3546
503-524-9318
www.nutritionforkids.com

Cover, Design & Illustration: Carol Buckle
Typesetting: Joan Pinkert
Editing: Andrea Howe

Printed in the United States of America

10 9 8 7

Library of Congress Control Number: 2003095564

Publisher's Cataloging in Publication

Evers, Connie Liakos.
    How to teach nutrition to kids / by Connie Liakos Evers.
    p. cm.
    Includes bibliograpical references and index.
    "This resource promotes positive attitudes about food, fitness and body image. Features hundreds of fun, hands-on nutrition education activities aimed at children ages 6-12."
    LCCN 2003095564
    ISBN 0-9647970-1-1

    1. Nutrition—Study and teaching (Elementary)
  I. Title.

TX364.E957 2003   372.3'7'044
                         QB103-200656

To Mom and Dad, my biggest fans.

Thanks for teaching me about nutrition, gardening and the importance of family meals.

(Sorry about the picky eating.)

Acknowledgements

A big "Thanks" to:

Students of Beaverton and Portland schools who wrote funny, endearing and often revealing thank-you letters over the years, some of which are excerpted in the quotes that begin each chapter.

Carol Buckle, graphic designer and friend who, in addition to her marvelous design, cover art and illustrations, can always make me laugh.

Joan Pinkert, typesetter and cheerleader with the most impeccable attention to detail!

Jennifer Butler, a wonderful teacher who contributed the "Nutrition Notes" at the end of Chapter 3.

The many professionals who have helped me along the way: Bob Honson; Brenda Ponichtera, R.D.; Bridget Swinney, M.S., R.D.; Penny Price, M.S.; Sandy Miller, M.S., R.D. and Margaret Raker, J.D.

Scott, Kelli, Sam and Adam. Of course!

Table of Contents

Introduction

Food is much more than a vehicle for delivering nutrients — it is an integral part of our lives. From our first suckling of the breast until our very last meal, food never lingers far from our minds or activities. Food brings people together — for daily meals, wedding feasts, backyard cookouts, sporting events and just about every social occasion imaginable.

Nutrition is the science that explores the myriad of chemical reactions that occur inside the cells of our bodies. From the combustion of carbohydrate for energy to the use of protein to heal a paper cut to the building of bone in a growing child, nutrition in action is something we don't have to consciously think about.

But to supply the best raw materials for the elegant workings of our bodies, we must give *food* some thought. Eating habits and food memories are imprinted early on and difficult to change later, a fact many adults learn all too well when they attempt to alter lifelong eating behaviors.

The purpose of this book is to give educators, nutrition professionals, parents and other caregivers the tools they need to teach 6- to 12-year-old children about food and nutrition in a meaningful and integrated way. My hope is that children will learn to enjoy a variety of healthful foods, find pleasure in physical activity and feel satisfaction in their growing, developing bodies.

Ideas are drawn from my experience as a nutrition educator working with school districts and my job as a parent feeding three growing children. Along the way, I have learned a great deal about how to succeed in teaching nutrition to kids. I have also had a lot of fun doing it! I hope you share my enthusiasm and allow your own creativity to expand and build on the many ideas presented here.

How to Use This Book

A cooperative approach among caregivers is necessary if children are to both learn and practice good eating habits. Described below are suggestions on how those who care for and teach children can best incorporate ideas and activities from this book.

Educators

The chapters in this book bear little resemblance to a standard nutrition book. Take a look at the Table of Contents. Instead of chapters like "Vegetables," "Vitamins" or "Weight Control," you will see "Language Arts," "Math" and "Social Studies," the subjects teachers spend time on *every* day of the school year. Many of the lesson ideas are designed with time in mind — easy to implement with little preparation. Others can be modified for simplicity or expanded into a comprehensive unit. For instance, the gardening ideas in Chapter 7 could easily comprise a year-long theme.

Throughout this book, you can readily identify how nutrition lesson ideas cross over into other disciplines. The following picture symbols identify related subject areas:

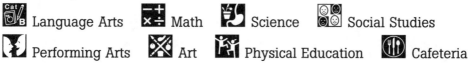

Language Arts   Math   Science   Social Studies

Performing Arts   Art   Physical Education   Cafeteria

Activities that require materials and supplies beyond what is commonly found in most classrooms are highlighted with **"You Will Need"** boxes. Activities are categorized according to level (primary, intermediate or either) in the index listing for each subject area.

Chapter 4, "Teaching the Basics of Healthful Eating," provides guidance on how to design your introductory nutrition unit, ideally taught early in the school year. Once students have a grasp of these basic concepts, you can expand and reinforce nutrition by integrating it into your curriculum all year long. As you plan your units of instruction and learning centers, keep this book handy. Refer to each subject area chapter as you plan lessons.

Many of the nutrition ideas may be the hook to get kids motivated in other subjects, too. Writing a letter to "Baby Bear," graphing food intake or analyzing the school lunch menu can make writing, math and critical thinking more exciting and relevant.

Before you plan lessons involving food preparation, please review Appendix A, "Guidelines for Safe Classroom Cooking."

Finally, take a look around your classroom. Are food and nutrition teaching materials up to date? If you have a kitchen, grocery store or restaurant as part of your dramatic play area, do the play foods include healthful choices? (An inexpensive way to update this area is to use real food packages, stuffed with pillow foam, if needed.)

Resources for low-cost materials that will brighten your classroom and reinforce nutrition concepts are listed in Appendix B.

Food/Nutrition Professionals

In nearly every chapter, students are encouraged to become involved with the school nutrition program. Examples include touring the school kitchen, writing letters to the school nutrition director, analyzing the school breakfast and lunch menus and performing lunchtime nutrition skits.

Just as nutrition is integrated into all subject areas, this book also gives guidance for integrating nutrition education into the school meal program. After all, the school cafeteria is the ultimate laboratory, giving students the chance to practice nutrition concepts each day.

Whenever possible, make yourself available to the teachers and students in your school. Volunteer to be a guest speaker on nutrition. Your presentation can be as simple as reading a storybook with a good-food message or as complicated as setting up a classroom sandwich bar to illustrate a meal that exemplifies the 2005 *MyPyramid*. This book provides hundreds of ideas on classroom nutrition lessons.

Another powerful way to reinforce nutrition concepts is to run promotions in the cafeteria. Menu or recipe contests, food-of-the-week displays, nutrition bingo with small incentives, student poster art and point-of-choice nutrition information encourage students to make healthful food choices. Chapter 12 provides guidance on how to turn the cafeteria into a center for nutrition education.

Parents

You are the ultimate gatekeeper of nutrition. What you buy, how you cook and the foods that *you* eat or refuse all send strong messages about food to your child. The best way to educate your child about nutrition and health is to model good eating behavior.

Beyond your role as food provider and living example, there are many other ways to teach your child about food and nutrition. A number of ideas in this book can easily be adapted for learning situations in the home. Tending a small garden plot, reading and discussing books with nutrition messages or using the grocery store as a learning center are just a few examples.

Involve your child in the kitchen. It's true that cooking with your child may add to the time, mess and confusion initially. But eventually, you will appreciate both the extra set of hands and your child's growing self-sufficiency.

Many of the food activities, especially the edible art creations in Chapter 10, work well in group settings such as birthday parties, scout meetings or large family gatherings.

This book can also serve as a stepping stone for initiating a nutrition education program in your local elementary school. Activities and ideas can be implemented by parent volunteers in the classroom or at school wellness, health, multicultural or science fairs. Information presented here also provides valuable guidance for setting school nutrition policy.

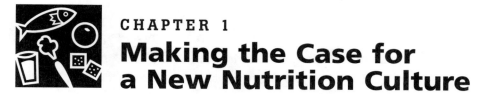

CHAPTER 1

Making the Case for a New Nutrition Culture

As parents and educators, it is our job to create a new culture for health, one where we model good eating and fitness habits, provide healthful shared meals and set limits on foods with little nutritional value.

A Great Need

Children today face an increasing number of nutrition problems, including fragmented eating habits, poor food choices, obesity and eating disorders. We are obviously failing to create an environment that is conducive to healthful eating and lifetime physical activity. Current findings shed a dim light on the state of children's eating and exercise habits.

OBESITY

Findings from the Center for Disease Control and Prevention (CDC) National Health and Nutrition Examination Survey document continued increase in the number of overweight children and teens. Sixteen percent of children and teens are considered overweight, a tripling of the level since 1980! An additional 15 percent of kids and teens are considered "at risk" for becoming overweight (defined by a body mass index between the 85th and 95th percentile).

Not only do these children face an uncertain future health picture, they are at risk right now for the debilitating effects of extra weight, such as high blood cholesterol levels, high blood pressure, low self-esteem and an increased risk of type 2 diabetes. This epidemic increase in childhood overweight is particularly prevalent among African American and Hispanic children, with more than 21 percent of these groups meeting the classification of overweight. It is estimated that about half of overweight school-agers and 70 percent of overweight teens of will remain obese into adulthood.

INACTIVITY

A big contributor to this trend is our fixation on all things electronic. Kids spend large chunks of passive time in front of the television, video games and computers. Studies have documented a clear connection between the time spent watching TV and the levels of both body fat and blood cholesterol in kids.

Besides increasing the temptation to snack on advertised foods, television has replaced active play for many kids. While the CDC and other organizations recommend that children participate in physical activity a minimum of an hour daily, kids are actually engaging in *less* physical activity, particularly as they approach adolescence. Nearly half of American youths ages 12–21 are not vigorously active on a regular basis.

POOR FOOD CHOICES

With a food supply as plentiful and varied as we have in the United States, it is shocking to note the dismal state of children's (and adults'!) food choices. Most children have a diet that "needs improvement," according to the Healthy Eating Index (HEI), a scale that measures 10 components of a healthful diet. As children move from preschool through adolescence, HEI scores decrease from an average of 75.7 for 2- to 3-year-olds to around 60 for teenagers. (An overall score of 80 is considered a "good" diet.)

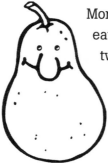

More than 75 percent of children ages 6–11 do not eat the minimum of three servings of vegetables or two servings of fruit daily. Of the vegetables eaten by children, approximately 55–65 percent come from either potatoes or tomatoes. Children have especially low intakes of the nutrient-rich dark green leafy and deep yellow vegetables and nutrient-dense citrus fruits, melon and berries.

Few youngsters take in enough calcium to maximize their lifetime bone development. At a time when they need calcium the most, kids are choosing soft drinks over dairy products and potato chips over broccoli. While recent government recommendations advise a calcium intake of 1,300 milligrams for children ages 9–18, nutrition surveys show a decline in calcium intake for this age group, with fewer than half consuming the recommended amount each day.

While snacking can contribute important nutrients to a child's diet, studies show that snacks are often a source of high-calorie, low-nutrient foods such as soft drinks, fried chips and sweet snacks. Total daily calorie intake from snacks among children has risen from an average of 450 to 600 calories per day over the past two decades, according to researchers at the University of North Carolina at Chapel Hill.

THE SUPER-SIZING OF AMERICA

It's no coincidence that we've seen a dramatic increase in the size of both food portions and our waistlines in recent years. For just a few more cents, we can stuff in more food, beverages and calories.

It's not just our imaginations — researchers have documented that the size of food portions are increasing. Using data from government food intake surveys, one study showed that portion sizes in restaurants *and* at home are increasing at an alarming rate.

Simply put, larger portions translate into more calories. Researchers have shown that even as early as age five, children will eat more when presented with larger portion sizes.

LIQUID CALORIES

"Got pop?" seems to be the real slogan for today's kids. Over the past twenty years, soft drink guzzling has soared among kids, while intake of milk and 100 percent fruit juice has taken a dive. This tendency to pick soda pop over more nutritious beverages actually begins in the early preschool years. By the time kids reach the teen years, nearly a fourth are downing more than 26 ounces of soft drinks daily.

One study documented that when children consumed an average of 9 ounces of soft drinks daily, their total daily calories increased, while key nutrients such as folate, vitamin A, vitamin C and calcium took a nosedive.

These liquid calories are not just coming from soft drinks — there has been a tremendous increase in sweetened beverage choices. Grocery store shelves overflow with bottles of sweetened nonjuice fruit drinks, teas and sports beverages.

HUNGRY CHILDREN

How can the same overnourished nation described here possibly have people who go hungry? It is shocking but true that hunger and inadequate nutrition continue to impact a startling number of children in America. A government report released in 2002 indicates that more than 16 percent of households with children are considered "food insecure," meaning they do not always have access to enough food for active, healthy lives for all household members.

Hungry children often fail to achieve their full academic potential. Children with inadequate diets are sick more, less active, less able to think and concentrate and more irritable and anxious. In one study, 6- to 11-year-old food-insufficient children had lower arithmetic scores and were more likely to have repeated a grade, have seen a psychologist and have had difficulty getting along with other children. Kids with iron deficiency anemia score lower on IQ tests (especially in vocabulary) and suffer from perceptual difficulties and low achievement.

One partial solution to this problem is better promotion of the school breakfast and lunch programs. Children who eat school meals, regardless of income level, have higher intakes of key nutrients and perform better in school.

Opportunity for Change

The news about children's health is not all bad. On the upside, a tremendous amount of interest, effort and opportunity currently surrounds this problem.

THE POWER OF PARENTS

Parents still have considerable influence over the eating patterns of their children. Studies point to a strong association between parents who model good nutrition and improved eating habits in their youngsters.

Kids and teens who eat meals with their families on a more frequent basis have higher intakes of several nutrients, including fiber, calcium, folate, iron and vitamins B6, B12, C and E.

Parents are also important partners in their children's nutrition education outside of the home. School-based nutrition programs that involve parents are more effective at changing children's eating behaviors than those that focus solely on the student.

KIDS IN THE KITCHEN

As children become more self-reliant at an earlier age, a "teachable moment" exists for strengthening food-related life skills.

Children who don't know how to cook often rely on fast foods or convenience foods of questionable nutritional quality. For this growing number of young consumers, nutrition education can really work when concepts are practical and applied, emphasizing skills such as shopping, label reading and cooking. Kids who are on their own for meals can immediately translate their nutrition knowledge into healthful eating behavior.

SCHOOL MEALS

Schools participating in the United States Department of Agriculture (USDA) child nutrition program are required to serve meals that meet the U.S. Dietary Guidelines for Americans. Unfortunately, kids don't always choose a balanced meal at school. Competition from vending machines, school stores and snack bars impede the integrity and intent of the school meal program. In an effort to raise money for school sports and other programs, we have unthinkingly sold out our children's health. Clearly, there is a great need for schools to create a more healthful environment (see Chapter 12).

EDUCATION

When educators realize that well-nourished students learn better, they are more inclined to move beyond the basic food groups and teach nutrition in a comprehensive, behavior-oriented manner.

A report from the National Center for Education Statistics in 2000 found that while 88 percent of elementary school teachers reported teaching nutrition in the classroom, not nearly enough time was devoted to nutrition education during the year. The mean number of hours spent on nutrition instruction was 13, well below the 50 hours thought to be necessary for impact on behavior.

Success at classroom nutrition education requires that teachers have sufficient background, training, resources and, of course, the time to teach it all! One goal of this book is to aid teachers in integrating nutrition across the curriculum and into the daily lives of students.

A Call to Action

Clearly, the efforts of many are needed to reverse the trends set forth here. The messages children receive about nutrition should be clear, consistent and constant. Only then will kids begin to internalize the information and make changes in their eating and activity habits. This formidable task of creating a healthful food culture is shared by all who influence kids' food choices: parents, extended family, educators, coaches, food/nutrition professionals, health care providers, researchers, the food industry, the media and legislators.

Most important, the food available to children must match the messages they are hearing. Whether at school, home, the ballpark or a restaurant, healthful choices that appeal to kids are essential. Kids don't get proficient at playing the piano, solving math problems or scoring soccer goals without a lot of practice — the same is true of good nutrition habits!

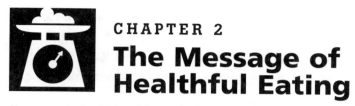

CHAPTER 2

The Message of Healthful Eating

If we are to instill healthy attitudes about food and body image in our children, we must start early, presenting a unified message about food as fuel and bodies as something to be proud of and happy about.

Finding a Balance

MEDIA MESSAGES

Presenting a balanced picture of nutrition is no easy task in today's society. The media confuses us daily, reporting the latest nutrition study as fact, leaving us dazed as we contemplate whether our favorite foods have been praised or denounced this week. We quickly lose sight that food really is enjoyable, necessary and sustains our lives!

Likewise, children are sent a mind-boggling set of mixed messages from television, the Internet and print media. On one hand, they see mostly "beautiful" people — at least by Hollywood or Madison Avenue's standard — who are thin, rich, popular and fun-loving. On the other hand, they are barraged with advertisements for foods with little nutritional value. When they do see the beautiful people eating, it is usually for ads that peddle foods such as candy, fried snacks and soft drinks.

Long before kids can read or write, they are influenced by advertising messages. In addition to the 30,000 TV ads each year aimed at the youth market, companies also reach children through in-school promotions, kids' clubs, cross-selling and other promotions, according to reports published by Consumers Union.

Food and beverages are the most advertised products on television programming aimed at kids. Most of these products are high in fat and/or sugar and of low nutritional value. Adding to the confusion, many ads directed at kids are deceptive in their nature. For instance, breakfast cereals and nonjuice beverages with "fruit" or "fruity" in their names are depicted in ads that include colorful images of real fruit. In actuality, many of the products contain no fruit or juice, relying on artificial flavors and colors for their "fruitiness."

While advertisers may be satisfied to know that their messages are working, the ultimate outcome of their efforts is detrimental to children's health. Studies show that there is a direct association between the number of hours of television viewed and the number of requests from children to buy the products they see advertised. Kids who watch the most TV have higher intakes of calories, fat, fried snacks, sweets and soft drinks and lower intakes of fruits and vegetables.

Even the youngest children are being swayed by marketers. In an experiment to test the impact of television commercials on the food preferences of 2- to 6-year-olds, researchers found that brief embedded commercials in a cartoon videotape directly influenced the preschoolers' food choices.

ALTERED BODY IMAGE

Not only is our society getting fatter, we also feel more guilty about it, a feeling children are acquiring at an alarmingly young age. In a study of 10- and 11-year-old Girls Scouts, 29 percent of the girls were trying to lose weight. More than 60 percent of fourth grade girls in an Iowa study reported a desire to be thinner. By age 18, nine out of ten teenage girls in a California survey were dieting to lose weight.

This perception of fatness is common even among girls with little body fat. In one study, 58 percent of girls ages 9 to 18 thought of themselves as fat, whereas only 15 percent were overweight based on height and weight measures. Fear of fatness, restrained eating and binge eating were found to be common among girls by age 10.

Boys may also have a disturbed body image, but their orientation is often toward a bigger and more muscular physique.

Parents have a powerful influence on their children's self-esteem and body image. Researchers found that measured self-esteem scores of kids ages 9–11 were lowered when they thought their parents were dissatisfied with their bodies. In boys, a lowered self-esteem was linked with both thinness and being perceived as too thin by parents. Not surprisingly, lowered self-esteem in girls had more to do with parental attitudes toward fatness. According to a 2000 study published in the Journal of the American Dietetic Association, moms who constantly diet directly influence their 5-year-old daughters' ideas about dieting.

Adding to the image problem is a small but worrisome group of overzealous parents. Determined that their child will not be fat or eat fat, they restrict food intake starting at a very young age. Kids who comply with their parents' wishes often end up underweight and at risk for delayed growth. Those who rebel may end up overweight because they have a tendency to overeat whenever they get the chance.

There is a wide variation in growth patterns and rates among kids. Children of the same age can vary as much as 40 pounds and 10 inches and still be considered "normal" by growth standards. Unfortunately, kids don't see a wide variety of shapes and sizes depicted in magazines or television. Even their school textbooks carry a "size bias." An analysis of third-grade texts since the beginning of the century found that illustrations of girls became increasingly thinner through the years, while no change was noted for pictures of boys.

Warning: Fashion Magazines May Make You Feel Bad!

Girls who read fashion magazines are more likely to go on diets. When researchers surveyed 548 5th–12th grade girls, they found that 69 percent of the girls reported that magazine models influenced their image of a perfect female body and 47 percent wanted to lose weight because of the magazine pictures.

Source: Field AE, Cheung L, Wolf AM, Herzog DB, Gortmaker SL, Colditz GA. Exposure to the mass media and weight concerns among girls. Pediatrics. 1999;103(3):E36.

Creating Positive Attitudes

Reversing the trend of feeling guilty about food and weight, resulting in indulgence, more weight and more guilt, can only be arrested through education and self-awareness.

If we are to instill healthy attitudes about food and body image in our children, we must start early, presenting a unified message about food as fuel and bodies as something to be proud of and happy about.

Now the hard part: we, as adult role models, must reach some degree of satisfaction with ourselves! Women, in particular, spend enormous amounts of time and energy pursuing that elusive ideal of a "perfect" body. In our constant obsession to diet, exercise and engage in dubious weight loss practices, we often forget that our basic body shape was predetermined at birth!

It's no wonder we're confused. In our lifetime alone, we have seen the "ideal" female body form go from voluptuous to outright undernourished! In an analysis of Miss America Pageant winners, researchers observed a drop in the Body Mass Index (BMI) over time. Only 23 percent of the winners had a BMI in the normal range of 20–25, and 26 percent actually met the World Health Organization's definition of undernourished (BMI < 18.5).

WHAT WE CAN DO

Despite the influence of popular culture, there are steps we can take to instill healthy attitudes in our children:

▲ Affirm children. When kids complain about being too fat, skinny, short, tall or slow, emphasize the goodness about them. Assure kids that people come in all different colors, shapes and sizes. Every child has a unique pattern of growth and will enter "growth spurts" at different times. Remind kids that there is no one "best" way to look.

▲ Children who you suspect are overweight should be referred to a qualified health care provider for evaluation and treatment. Often, counseling of an overweight child requires cooperation and participation by the entire family and school community.

▲ Emphasize the enjoyable aspects of food. Avoid labeling food as either medicine or poison. With older children especially, telling them "it's good for you" may actually discourage healthful eating habits. Likewise, kids are not immediately concerned that a food they like may clog their arteries or decay their teeth. Scare tactics rarely work.

▲ Children should have a choice over their eating and control over their bodies. Given a selection of healthful foods, kids have an amazing ability to self-regulate their diet. In spite of good intentions, adults impair the development of normal eating habits when they attempt to control a child's food intake.

Taken to extremes, an overcontrolling parent places a child at risk for developing eating disorders such as obesity, bulimia and anorexia nervosa.

Parents' Actions, Not Words, Key to Better Nutrition for Kids

If parents ate more fruits and vegetables, so did their daughters, researchers found in a study of 200 5-year-old girls and their parents.

Parents who pressured their daughters the most about eating fruits and vegetables were those who consumed the least of these foods. Their daughters ate 1.6 fewer servings of fruits and vegetables a day than the daughters of parents who used less pressure.

The researchers recommend that parents set a good example by eating plenty of fruits and vegetables and by not nagging.

Source: Fisher JO, Mitchell DC, Smiciklas-Wright H, Birch LL. Parental influences on young girls' fruit and vegetable, micronutrient, and fat intakes. J Am Diet Assoc. 2002;102:58-64.

▲ Encourage children to move, play and exercise, both at home and at school. Besides physical education and recess time, kids (and teachers!) can benefit from discovery classroom walks (see Chapter 11).

At home kids will gravitate toward more activity if they are regularly "unplugged" from television, computer and video games. Parents also reap benefits from family walks, bike rides and other shared activities.

▲ Make mealtime a priority. Breaking bread together promotes good nutrition habits. School-aged children who eat alone in front of the television tend to overeat, while younger children tend to eat fewer nutritious foods when isolated at meals.

Mealtime means more than refueling kids with nutrients — they also get a hefty dose of emotional, intellectual and spiritual nourishment. As families pass the peas and pour the milk, they also convey values and establish traditions.

Pay attention to the school mealtime atmosphere, too. Work to improve nutrition, taste, presentation and the overall mealtime atmosphere at school. Bright cafeterias, short lines and adequate time for children to eat should be goals of every school. Kids should be allowed to relax and socialize — these skills are also components of learning and development. Schools with limited facilities may want to explore "family-style" eating in the classroom.

What Kids Need to Know

Clearly, children are in desperate need of a balanced, sensible message about eating and nutrition. One goal of nutrition education is to enlighten and empower kids so they will grow to be adults who make informed food choices and avoid the lure of food fads and nutrition hype.

What then, should we be teaching kids? The following points outline the basic goals of nutrition education for kids. Chapters 4–12 provide specific, hands-on activities for reaching these goals.

▲ Emphasize food as it relates to life today. You will lose kids' attention faster than they can say "osteoporosis" if too much emphasis is placed on how proper nutrition prevents disease. If you succeed in reaching them with the good nutrition message today, their tomorrows will likely be healthier, too.

Remind children that healthful food promotes achievement. In school or on the playing field, kids who eat well perform better and achieve higher levels of mastery. A nutritious diet fuels the body for learning, growth, sports and play.

Well-nourished kids look better, too! Children who eat a balanced diet have eyes that sparkle, skin that glows and bodies that are fit and energetic.

▲ The message of good nutrition is summed up in the *Dietary Guidelines for Americans (2005 DGA)*. Adults and kids over the age of two are advised to aim for fitness through regular physical activity and moderate eating, balance their diets by eating from a wide selection of foods, emphasizing whole grains, fruits, vegetables, lean protein and low-fat dairy foods, and to choose sensibly by moderating the amount of fat, sugar and sodium they eat. The *DGA* offers simple advice that requires continued diligence to form into lifetime habits.

Revised every five years, the DGA are designed to help Americans choose diets that will meet nutrient requirements, promote health, support active lives and reduce risks of chronic disease. The DGA also guide U.S. food policies that affect nutrition programs such as USDA's School Meal and Food Stamp Programs, and the WIC Program (Supplemental Food Program for Women, Infants and Children). Published jointly by the United States Department of Agriculture (USDA) and the Department of Health and Human Services (HHS), the guidelines form the basis of the 2005 *MyPyramid* (see chapter 4 for more about *MyPyramid*).

For more information and educational materials, visit *www.healthierus.gov/dietaryguidelines*

Two important practical tools for meeting the DGA are *MyPyramid* and the *Nutrition Facts* food label. A "picture" of what a healthful diet looks like, *MyPyramid* is especially useful as a teaching aid for children. The *Nutrition Facts* label is a simplified, yet effective, device for analyzing foods and comparing their nutrient contents. Ideas for developing a nutrition unit around the *MyPyramid* and nutrition labels are included, respectively, in Chapters 4 and 6.

▲ Teach children to refuel their bodies! Because of their smaller stomach capacity and tremendous energy needs, kids require frequent meals and snacks. Behavior problems at times are merely the result of an empty stomach.

Breakfast is the meal most directly connected to school achievement. Kids who skip breakfast have shorter attention spans, do poorly in tasks requiring concentration and even score lower on standard achievement tests.

When researchers compared the diets of children who regularly eat breakfast with those who don't, they found that the breakfast skippers never fully compensate for the missed meal throughout the day. Children who ate a morning meal took in far more nutrients over the course of the day than those who missed breakfast.

Somehow, "snacking" has taken on a negative connotation in our society, perhaps because it is often linked with low-nutrient foods. Done right, snacks can and do make a big contribution to daily nutrition. Healthful snacks should mirror meals — emphasizing healthful foods, but in smaller quantities.

▲ Young bodies need to move! Nutrition studies show that the current epidemic of childhood obesity stems from both inactivity and overeating. An intricate balance exists between food and physical activity. A nutrition unit will be decidedly lacking if it fails to present the exercise part of the equation.

Kids enjoy learning about nutrition when it is presented from a fitness perspective. That's why Chapter 11 is devoted to nutrition as a component of the physical education curriculum. Physical fitness should also be part of the daily classroom routine, especially in schools that limit PE to once or twice weekly.

▲ Media literacy should be a part of every child's education, both at school and at home. If children are to resist the allure of the media, advertisements and other societal influences, they must learn to identify the intent of the messages. Even very young children can grasp the basic purpose of advertising (to sell us stuff!). Older children will enjoy homework they really can do in front of the TV, i.e., analyze and critique food ads.

Role playing is a very effective way to teach children the messages of the media and encourage the development of critical thinking and decision-making skills. Chapter 9 outlines several strategies for helping children to analyze and re-create the food messages they hear each day from TV, radio, magazines and peers.

Media Literacy Resources

American Academy of Pediatrics, Media Matters: National Media Education Campaign, *www.aap.org/advocacy/mediamatters.htm*

New Mexico Media Literacy Project, *http://www.nmmlp.org*

TV Turnoff Network, *www.tvturnoff.org*

CHAPTER 3

The F.I.B. Approach to Nutrition Education

"Thank you for the very tasty lesson — and the good yogurt with blueberries, bananas, strawberries and granola. Combined to make a masterpiece." —Jeremy

There was little in my training to become a registered dietitian that prepared me to teach nutrition to kids. In college, I spent my time learning the scientific basis of nutrition and key principles of food management. Not that the zinc requirement of rodents or hospital trayline efficiency weren't important issues, it's just that I failed to grasp the *practical* issues at the heart of feeding and teaching kids.

I wasn't sure what to do when kids decorated the wall with their spaghetti or nicknamed coconuts "dog poop balls" or stuffed peas up their noses.

And worse, I was guilty of boring kids to sleep by lecturing them about food groups!

In my position as the nutrition education coordinator for a large urban school district, I gained insight from those around me — teachers, parents, foodservice staff and *especially* the kids. I came to realize that key elements were often missing from efforts at nutrition education.

Boiled down to three words, the ingredients I discovered necessary for effective nutrition education with children are **Fun, Integrated** and **Behavioral**. Hence the acronym F.I.B. (though I certainly don't advocate lying!).

Make It Fun!

Like it or not, today's kids are easily bored. Products of the dot-com and video age, they are used to information that is entertaining, fast-paced and exciting. In a word, "fun."

Teachers increasingly need to engage as well as educate students. While this approach can mean more planning, the payoff is a boost in motivation. Children who enjoy themselves through discovery and experimentation are much more apt to listen and retain information.

Educators who create engaging lessons often enjoy their jobs more, too! During my career as a nutrition educator, I have:

▲ Appeared in classrooms around Halloween as "Nutra the Witch," teaching kids how to make "food group brew," choose healthful snacks and limit their candy "goblin."

▲ Acted in noontime nutrition shows for elementary schools with two full-sized dog characters named Sheggy Good-Grub and Sickly Spot. Sheggy's nickname was SHEG, an acronym for the four things nutrition gives a young body — strength, health, energy and growth. I even led the cafeteria in a round of "The Sheggy Good-Grub Song," in spite of dubious vocal skills. (Once, it was even broadcast on CNN!)

▲ Used my own baby as a "visual aid." Frustrated with my inability to reach teen moms, I brought my 10-month-old son along to demonstrate techniques for infant feeding. It was fun and also very effective!

▲ Developed *Crazy for Veggies* and *Go Bananas for Fruit* kits consisting of interactive worksheets, stickers and tasting/preparation ideas in order to motivate children to include more fruits and vegetables in their diets.

▲ Sang, danced, exercised, cooked and led puppet shows with elementary school kids more times than I can count!

THINK BIG!

When planning a nutrition lesson or entire unit, brainstorm creative ways to make the concepts come alive. Say, for example, kids are routinely feeding their oranges to the trash during lunch. Your goal is to encourage kids to eat (or at least try) oranges.

Talking about oranges is boring. Putting up colorful posters of oranges throughout the school is a little better. Providing cut up oranges for snacks is better still.

But to really make an impact, declare one day "Orange Day." Serve orange juice on the breakfast menu and orange wedges at lunch. Encourage students, staff and visiting parents to wear orange, call the citrus commission to see if they have teaching materials (and maybe even an orange costume to lend) and set up centers where students can make orange juice, plant the seeds from their oranges or write a story about oranges. Ask parents to send favorite recipes using oranges or orange juice. Decorate the cafeteria with student-made "Orange you glad you eat oranges?" posters. The ideas are endless.

Overkill? Perhaps. But this example illustrates how one nutrition concept — oranges are a tasty and healthful food — can be integrated into the entire school environment. Students pick up skills in science (making orange juice and planting seeds), language arts (writing a story) and art (making posters). Staff, parents and the school cafeteria all become involved, too, making this an integrated effort. Which leads us to the next letter of "F.I.B."

Integrate Nutrition Wherever Possible

Success with nutrition education largely depends on how well it is integrated into other subject areas, intertwined with the school cafeteria and reinforced through food experiences at home.

With barely enough time to teach kids the core subjects such as math and reading, teachers struggle to find time to teach nutrition. It's not that educators aren't interested in nutrition. In a survey of Connecticut teachers, 98 percent of elementary teachers felt that nutrition should be taught in school, but only 56 percent reported teaching nutrition to their students.

Lack of teacher training is also a barrier to nutrition education. Only about half of teachers have had formal training to teach nutrition, according to a 2000 report from the National Center for Education Statistics.

While teachers prefer to integrate nutrition into other subject areas, they don't always have the time or skills to accomplish this goal. Studies show that when nutrition is an integral part of the school day, teachers teach more nutrition over the course of the year than when they present it as a separate unit.

THE CAFETERIA

Once thought of as a necessary distraction, the school nutrition program is gaining respect as an adjunct to the education of students. As they serve kids breakfast and lunch, nutrition staff who receive proper training can also be enlisted to serve good-nutrition messages.

As school nutrition directors strive to plan kid-accepted menus that meet the *Dietary Guidelines for Americans*, strive for universal meals and meet the nutritional needs of chronically ill children, their success will depend on the strength of their integration with the classroom and school community.

To be truly effective, the food and messages received in the school cafeteria should complement nutrition instruction by teachers. A solid nutrition education program in the classroom will confuse and dismay students if they are faced with a display of high-fat, low-nutrient fare in the cafeteria. Likewise, making healthful meal changes without teaching students, parents and school staff the rationale behind the menu switch will likely result in a lot of grumbling and a drop in cafeteria sales.

Chapter 12 is devoted to making the cafeteria a center for nutrition education.

TAKING THE MESSAGE HOME

It is essential to link nutrition education to the home environment. Through parent meetings, interaction with parent-teacher groups, newsletters, menus and information sent home, good nutrition concepts can be reinforced. Parents have a lot to contribute, too! Joining their children at school meals, setting up health and nutrition "fairs," assisting with classroom nutrition lessons, volunteering in the school kitchen or cafeteria or selling *nutritious* foods as a fundraiser for education projects are important ways parents can become involved in school nutrition.

Since the bulk of purchasing, food preparation and eating happens at home, kids may need to serve as nutrition teachers, too, encouraging parents to buy and try new foods and experiment with different cooking methods. Assigning cooking "homework" is one way to get the family (and maybe even the dog) involved.

Table 3-1

EFFECTIVE NUTRITION EDUCATION: WHAT THE RESEARCH SHOWS

According to a report published in the *Journal of Nutrition Education*, the following components contribute to successful nutrition education with elementary-aged students:

- Instruction with a behavioral focus (better to focus on changing specific behaviors rather than on just learning nutrition facts)
- Use of active learning strategies (not just lectures)
- Devotion of adequate time and intensity to nutrition education (the time needed to impact attitudes and behavior is estimated at 50 hours per year)
- A family involvement component
- School meals and food-related policies that reinforce classroom nutrition education
- Teachers with adequate training in nutrition education

Source: Lytle, LA. Nutrition Education for School-Aged Children. J Nutr Ed, 1995; 27 (6): 298-311.

Emphasize Behavior Change

Nutrition is not just another "subject." Like health or physical education, the goal reaches beyond the acquisition of knowledge. Ultimately, we want to produce changes in the daily eating behavior of children. As the example above illustrates, knowing oranges are nutritious isn't enough — eating more oranges is the ultimate goal.

Behavior change does not happen quickly, particularly in adults. It is a process — an evolution that requires a cycle of attempts and failures to finally succeed. That is why some smokers quit and start many times before finally quitting. Or those seeking a slimmer figure lose, plateau, gain and lose weight over and over again.

Fortunately, it is easier to produce nutrition and health behavior change in children. Especially before age 12, children are much more likely to take concepts they learn and put them to practice. In a Minnesota study that tracked children from grade six through adolescence, kids who learned to make positive health decisions in regard to smoking, physical activity and food choices prior to sixth grade ended up with healthier habits as teens. An encouraging follow-up to the CATCH (Child and Adolescent Trial for Cardiovascular Health) Study found that three years after their last formal exposure to vigorous physical activity and nutrition lessons, the eighth graders continued to practice many of the heart-healthy behaviors they had learned in elementary school.

However, teaching nutrition once a year as a unit, regardless of intensity, will have little impact on long-term behavior change. Those concepts need to be reinforced all year, for many years, to make appreciable changes.

Lessons aimed at behavior change have two things in common: 1) real experience with food and 2) a real-life, reachable goal. Research done with Cookshop, a food-based nutrition education program based in New York, showed that when the curriculum included cooking in the classroom, students ate more of the same foods (grains and vegetables) served in the cafeteria.

For instance, a lesson about grains might include a bread baking (and eating) activity and end by encouraging students to eat at least six servings each day. Devising a chart to check off how many grains are eaten gives students a chance to sharpen math skills. Homework could consist of a simple muffin or granola recipe for the students to try with their families. The school cafeteria might highlight the foods made from grain that week, even including a few new ones such as couscous or quinoa. Again, this is an example of an integrated approach to nutrition education aimed at behavior change.

Table 3-2

NUTRITION NOTES
FROM A FIFTH GRADE TEACHER

In February our class took a good look at our daily eating habits. Each student kept a record of what he or she ate for four days. Students discovered that they had some nutritional holes! Many students were not eating enough grains, vegetables and fruits.

Students set goals to try to eat more food from the food group in which they weren't getting enough servings. They then kept a record of their eating habits for four more days. The results? Most students improved their eating habits. All students became more aware of how many servings per day they should have of each kind of food and what it means to eat a balanced diet.

We learned about how eating a balanced diet can help improve our health, and which foods contain nutrients such as vitamin C, potassium and calcium. We also learned that eating a breakfast made up of foods from at least three food groups can help them do better in school!

A healthful snack of food from at least two food groups can help boost their energy and concentration during the school day. For snack time, students are encouraged to bring healthful snacks, and now, most do. Many of the kids in our classroom are involved in sports or physical play after school. Connie Evers, a registered dietitian (and Sam's mom), came into our classroom to show us how to eat healthfully for athletic activities. We learned that active bodies need carbohydrates to help them stay full of energy. Students also learned that drinking water before, during and after an athletic event is important. Mrs. Evers showed us how to make fruit garnishes out of kiwi and strawberries. Yum!

Students made posters for the cafeteria encouraging other students in our school to eat a well-balanced meal.

Source: Jennifer (Hansen) Butler, Hansen's Headlines, parent newsletter, March 2001.

The Bottom Line

Perhaps the best case for promoting good eating behavior is the immediate effects it has on learning and development. A child who is hungry or poorly nourished is not ready to learn. Nutrition education done right is a boost for education in general. Practicing good nutrition habits makes kids better learners of *all* subjects.

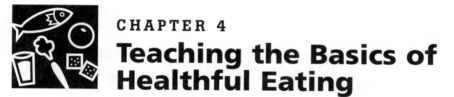

CHAPTER 4

Teaching the Basics of Healthful Eating

"I've been cooking for my family for years, and I've always made well-balanced meals with every food group." —Allison, age 10

Grasping the concept of food groups has long been a goal of nutrition education. While the food groups have changed names, number and emphasis over the years, the basic principles have remained the same: We need to eat different kinds of foods in varying amounts to keep our bodies functioning at full capacity. The three keywords often used to describe the food group system are *variety*, *balance* and *moderation*.

Nutrition scientists continue to study and discover the most optimal diet that contributes to lifelong health. To reflect this knowledge, the United States Department of Agriculture (USDA) introduced the *Dietary Guidelines for Americans 2005* (*www.healthierus.gov/dietaryguidelines*) and a new corresponding food guide a few months later. Termed *MyPyramid: Steps to a Healthier You*, the emphasis is on individual food needs and physical activity. The biggest change? The graphic is now more of a symbol or icon — not a detailed food guide — and directs users to *www.MyPyramid.gov* for specific advice on eating plans and exercise.

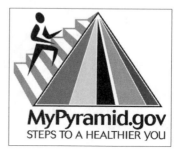

MyPyramid for Kids is a simplified version of *MyPyramid* with kid-friendly graphics and the slogan "Eat right. Exercise. Have fun." Targeted to 6-to 11-year-olds, posters, work-sheets, games and lessons are available at

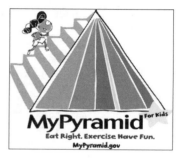

www.MyPyramid.gov/kids. A colored poster of *MyPyramid for Kids* is featured on the inside back cover of this book.

Table 4-1

Highlights of *MyPyramid*

▲ PHYSICAL ACTIVITY

For the first time, a symbol of physical activity is an integral part of the food guide. While the link between activity and nutrition has long been recognized, this graphic is one more reminder that food and fitness are partners in good health. Children should strive to be physically active at least 60 minutes each day.

▲ FOOD GROUP NAMES & MESSAGES

Each vertical band of *MyPyramid* represents a different food group (and an additional small stripe represents oils, which is not technically a food group). The vertical bands vary in width according to the approximate proportion that the food group should contribute to the diet. The names of the food groups have been simplified and each group is paired with a key message. The new names/messages are:

- Grains — Make half your grains whole.
- Vegetables — Vary your veggies.
- Fruits — Focus on fruits.
- Milk — Get your calcium-rich foods.
- Meat & Beans — Go lean with protein.

The poster on the inside back cover features the *MyPyramid* groups in color along with their labels and messages.

▲ SERVING SIZES

Americans have long struggled with making sense of serving sizes. Our ever-growing portions have contributed to our expanding waistlines. In an effort to relate more effectively to Americans, servings are now listed in U.S. household measurements such as cups and ounces.

Refer to Table 4–2 for more information on serving sizes and recommendations for children (for adults, you can visit *www.MyPyramid.gov* for this information).

▲ EMPHASIS ON WHOLE GRAINS

New to *MyPyramid* is a prescription for the amount of whole grains to include each day. The advice is simple — make half your grains whole. Whole grains are nutritionally superior to their refined counterparts. Because they contain the entire grain kernel, whole grains possess more fiber, vitamins, minerals and phytochemicals than grains that have had the outer covering and germ removed. A minimum of three servings of whole grains are recommended each day.

Examples of whole grains:

- Bulgur (cracked wheat) ▸ Brown Rice ▸ Oatmeal
- Stone-ground cornmeal or grits (not the degerminated varieties)
- Products made with 100 percent whole-wheat flour, such as breads, cereals, pasta, pancakes and waffles
- Cereals made from wheat bran (or that contain added wheat bran)

Table 4-1 (continued)

> **▲ EMPHASIS ON HEALTHFUL FAT SOURCES**
> Most nutrition experts agree that there is an advantage to choosing fats such as
> olive oil, canola oil, avocados, olives, nuts and fatty fish rather than the saturated
> fats found in animal products. Other fats known to raise cholesterol levels are the
> hydrogenated and partially hydrogenated fats (also known as trans fats) and
> saturated vegetable fats such as coconut oil and palm kernel oil. (See the dietary
> fat primer on pages 171–172.)
>
> **▲ DISCRETIONARY CALORIES**
> Replacing the old pyramid "tip" is a category that *MyPyramid* refers to as
> "discretionary calories." These refer to the calories left for sweets, treats and
> fats once nutrition needs are met with more healthful fare.
>
> *NOTE: To simplify this concept for children, this category will be referred to in this book as*
> *"extra" foods. Most children who eat a balanced diet can fit in 1-2 servings of "extra"*
> *foods each day. The trick, however, is to exercise portion control and to read and*
> *understand Nutrition Facts labels. Chips, candy, soft drinks, cookies and other "extras"*
> *often contain several servings in one package.*

HOW MUCH?

Table 4-2 provides information on the food groups, how much is needed
each day and examples of foods in each food group.

Teaching *MyPyramid*

Before you begin your basic nutrition unit, be sure to obtain a classroom-sized
poster for reference from *http://teachfree.org/onliMyPyramidPoster.aspx.*
You can also download colored posters and materials from
www.mypyramid.gov/kids.

CONCEPTS TO TEACH

The following points outline the key messages children should grasp when
studying *MyPyramid*.

▲ There are five different food groups and a small stripe that indicates oils
(oils are not considered an actual food group). The width of the food group
bands represent the approximate proportion of that food group in the diet.

Table 4-2

MyPyramid — Recommended needs for children ages 6–11

FOOD GROUP	AMOUNT NEEDED EACH DAY	EXAMPLES	GO EASY ON
Grains	5 to 7 ounces (more if you are extra active)	1 ounce is approximately: 1 slice of bread; 1 cup of dry cereal; 1/2 cup of rice, pasta or cooked cereal; 3 cups of popcorn; 1 small tortilla; 7 round crackers	Refined grains; Choose mostly whole grains
Vegetables	1-1/2 to 2-1/2 cups	1 cup cooked or chopped vegetables; 2 cups salad greens is considered 1 cup from the vegetable group	High-fat salad dressings, butter added to cooked vegetables and fried vegetables such as French fries
Fruits	1-1/2 cups	1 cup of fruit or 100% juice; Also equal to 1 cup of fruit: 1 small apple; 1 large banana; 1 large orange; 32 grapes; 1/2 cup dried fruit	Fruit with added sugar
Milk	2 cups (up to age 8) 3 cups (age 9 and older)	1 cup of milk or yogurt or 1-1/2 ounces of cheese	High-fat cheeses and high-sugar dairy desserts
Meat & Beans	4-6 ounces total of meat or meat equivalents	1 ounce lean meat, chicken or fish; 1/4 cup beans, 1 egg, 1 tablespoon of peanut butter, 1/2 ounce (about 2 tablespoons) of shelled sunflower seeds or nuts	High-fat meats

Limit "Extra" foods such as candy, chocolate, cookies, sweetened drinks and fried chips to 1 to 2 servings on most days.

▲ Each group provides certain nutrients that help our bodies work at their best. The body needs a total of about 40 nutrients, which fall into six general classes: **Carbohydrates, Protein, Fat, Vitamins, Minerals** and **Water**. Eating foods from all the food groups is one way to get the nutrients needed for good health (see Table 4–3).

In addition to the basic nutrients, there are also a whole host of beneficial chemicals in many foods that benefit the body in a variety of ways. Termed "phytochemicals" (translation: plant chemicals), these beneficial substances often protect body cells from damage. Foods with beneficial chemicals are also known as "functional foods." Table 4-4 provides some examples of specific phytochemicals found in various foods.

▲ We need the most servings of grains because they are rich in energy-giving carbohydrates and fiber. In addition, grains are rich in several B vitamins and iron. Our bodies' first and most important need is for energy. Besides the energy it takes for play and sports, we also use energy just to keep us alive. With each breath, heartbeat or blink of the eyes, we are "spending" energy.

Whole grains are superior to refined grains because they include additional fiber, vitamins, minerals and beneficial phytochemicals. Regular consumption of whole grains is important for digestive health, reduces the rate of coronary heart disease and decreases the risk of several types of cancer. Surveys show that most Americans are lucky to consume even one serving of whole grains daily. When children are offered whole grains beginning at a young age, they adapt to the coarser texture of whole-grain breads and cereals.

Fiber, while not exactly a nutrient, helps the body to move food through the digestive system. Fiber also helps our health in other ways, too (e.g., some fibers lower blood cholesterol and stabilize blood sugar levels). Whole grains such as brown rice and 100 percent whole-wheat bread

Table 4-3

NUTRIENTS AND WHAT THEY DO

FOOD GROUP	KEY NUTRIENTS*	ACTION IN THE BODY
Grains	Carbohydrate, Fiber, B vitamins, Iron	**Carbohydrate** is the body's major source of energy. **Fiber** aids the movement of food through the digestive tract. **B vitamins** help in the body's use of energy. **Iron** carries oxygen in red blood cells and muscle cells.
Vegetables	Vitamin A, Vitamin C, Folate, Iron, Magnesium, Fiber	**Vitamin A** helps maintain skin and mucous membranes and aids in vision. **Vitamin C** helps the the body heal and fight infections. **Folate** is needed for healthy blood cells and is important for cell division, such as in pregnancy and growth. **Magnesium** is found in bones and is important for muscle and nerve functioning.
Fruits	Vitamin A, Vitamin C, Potassium, Folate, Fiber	**Potassium** maintains the heart beat, regulates body fluids, and is needed for muscle and nerve functioning.
Meat & Beans	Protein, B vitamins, Iron, Zinc	**Protein** provides the building blocks needed for growth, replacement and maintenance of body tissues. Zinc is necessary for healing, taste perception, growth and sexual development.
Milk	Calcium, Vitamin D, Riboflavin, Potassium, Protein	**Calcium** is needed for the development and maintenance of healthy bones and teeth. **Vitamin D** is a partner with calcium in building and maintaining strong bones. **Riboflavin** is a B vitamin that helps the body use energy.
"Extras" (Not a food group)	Simple carbohydrates (sugars), Fat	**Simple carbohydrates** or sugars provide energy but few other nutrients. **Fat** is a source of energy and helps in the absorption of certain vitamins. More healthful fat choices include olive oil, canola oil, avocados, olives, nuts and fatty fish.

There are more than 40 different nutrients with many different functions that are required for good health. Each food group contributes many other nutrients in addition to the "key nutrients" listed here.

Table 4-4

PHYTOCHEMICALS IN OUR FOOD

While we have long understood that food provides essential nutrients, researchers now realize that hundreds of non-nutrient chemicals — collectively known as phytochemicals — may promote optimal health, protect body cells and lower the risk of chronic diseases such as cancer and cardiovascular disease.

Scientists are only beginning to unravel the questions of how they work, how much is needed to exert a protective effect and whether the chemicals work alone or in conjunction with other substances in a food.

The advice for today? Include a wide variety of healthful foods in your daily diet and the phytochemicals are sure to follow!

A Few Examples:

PHYTOCHEMICAL	POSSIBLE HEALTH BENEFITS	FOOD SOURCES
Anthocyanins	Antioxidant that may protect against effects of aging	Blueberries, plums, cherries, strawberries
Beta Glucan (soluble fiber)	Lowers blood cholesterol levels	Oats
Catechins	Reduces the risk of cancer	Black and green tea
Elagic Acid	Reduces the risk of cancer; lowers blood cholesterol levels	Red grapes, kiwifruit, blueberries, raspberries, strawberries, blackberries
Lutein	Promotes eye health (especially as we age)	Dark green leafy vegetables, kiwifruit, broccoli
Lycopene	Reduces the risk of prostate cancer and heart disease	Tomatoes, red pepper, pink grapefruit, watermelon
Omega-3 Fatty Acids	Reduces the risk for heart disease	Cold-water fish such as salmon, mackerel, herring and sardines; flaxseed oil; walnuts
Probiotics	Aids gastrointestinal health	Yogurt and other fermented dairy products
Sulforaphane	Reduces the risk of cancer	Broccoli, cauliflower, cabbage, Brussels sprouts
Sulfur Compounds	Reduces the risk of cancer; lowers blood cholesterol and blood pressure	Garlic, onions, chives, leeks, scallions

have more fiber than refined white rice or bread made from enriched flour. (Other fiber-rich foods include beans, fruits and vegetables.)

▲ The fruit and vegetable groups are important because they give us a whole host of vitamins, minerals, carbohydrates, fiber and phytochemicals. Children need approximately 1-1/2 cups of fruit and 1-1/2 to 2-1/2 cups of vegetables each day for good health and good looks, too! The vitamins, minerals and phytochemicals in fruits and vegetables also help keep our skin, eyes and hair healthy.

▲ Milk provides calcium, vitamin D, riboflavin, potassium, protein and many more nutrients. Kids ages 9 and older need 3 cups of low-fat or fat-free milk — or an equivalent amount of low-fat yogurt and/or low-fat cheese (1 cup yogurt or 1-1/2 ounces of cheese equals 1 cup of milk) — every day. For kids aged 2 to 8, it's 2 cups of milk or the equivalent.

What if you can't drink milk?

▲ If you are lactose intolerant, you can probably tolerate specially treated lactose-reduced milk, yogurt with active cultures or aged cheese such as cheddar.

▲ If you follow a vegetarian diet that includes no animal products (known as a vegan) or have a milk allergy, you need to include nondairy sources of calcium in your diet such as calcium-fortified soy or rice milk, calcium-set tofu, calcium-fortified fruit juices, broccoli, kale, almonds and calcium-fortified breakfast cereals.

▲ If you eat fish, calcium-rich sources include sardines and canned salmon (canned with the bones).

▲ The meat & beans group is rich in many nutrients, including protein, B vitamins, iron and zinc. Most children need around 4–6 ounces of meat or meat equivalents each day. To lower fat intake, choose lean meats, chicken without the skin, fish, beans and other low-fat meat alternates.

KNOWING HOW MUCH TO EAT

Most kids need to eat at least the minimum amount recommended from each food group. But many kids will need more, especially those who are active in sports and play. Here is one way to explain this to children:

How much you eat is entirely up to you. Well, at least it's up to your body. While dietitians can use complicated equations to figure out about how many calories you need for growth, activity and energy, they can also be wrong. That is because your body is a one-of-a-kind. You are growing and changing and your activity level is not always the same. Some days you need more calories and some days you need fewer.

The best way to know how much to eat is to listen to your body! Eat only when you are hungry (not bored or sad or frustrated) and only until your body feels comfortably full.

A rating scale like the one below can help you to learn how much to eat. It's best to eat when your stomach feels about like a "2" on the chart below and stop eating at "3." When you wait to eat until you are at "1," you may want to eat everything in sight. When you keep eating until "4" or "5," you can end up putting too much energy in your body, which will be stored as extra fat. The best way to know how much to eat is to listen to your body! Eat until your body feels comfortably full. You should feel satisfied but not overly stuffed.

ACTIVITY

HOW FULL ARE YOU?

Lead children in a discussion of how it feels to eat too much, not enough and just the right amount. Next, ask them to develop a rating scale for hunger and fullness, with 1 being really hungry and 5 being overstuffed (like Thanksgiving).

Example:

Starving!	My stomach feels empty.	I feel just right — not too hungry or too full.	I'm feeling too full.	I ate way too much! I don't feel so well.
1	2	3	4	5

For 1–3 days, ask them to use the scale to note their level of hunger/fullness before and after each meal. Ask them if they noticed any patterns. Are they eating about the right amount of food? Discuss how this assignment can help them to regulate their food to more closely match their bodies' needs.

AVOIDING *"MyPyramid* OVERLOAD"

Break *MyPyramid* concepts into several sessions so children can fully "digest" the material. Each session should ideally have a hands-on, discovery activity (see next section for ideas). Below is a suggested timeline for presenting information, although it will vary according to age and developmental level.

▲ **Session 1:** Introduce the *MyPyramid* poster and explain how foods for good health are divided into five main food groups. Plan activities that allow students to sort and categorize foods into the five food groups. Discuss how the vertical bands on the pyramid are different sizes and this means we need more servings from the groups with the widest bands.

▲ **Session 2:** Review the amounts suggested for each food group. Lead the class in discussion of "How much food do I need?" Set up measuring centers where students can discover the serving sizes of various foods.

▲ **Session 3:** Introduce the concept of nutrients and list the six classes (Carbohydrates, Protein, Fat, Vitamins, Minerals, Water). Explain that because each food group contains a different set of nutrients, we need foods from all the groups to get the nutrients our bodies need. Highlight how key nutrients are needed to build and maintain a healthy body (see Table 4-3). Discuss with older students the concept of the beneficial chemicals in food known as phytochemicals (see Table 4-4).

▲ **Session 4:** Ask the class for examples of low-nutrition "extra" foods that do not fit into any of the *MyPyramid* groups. Discuss the concept of dietary excess (e.g., how we need to limit foods that are high in sugar and fat) and the importance of eating these foods in moderation (i.e., limiting to 1-2 servings on most days).

Planning *MyPyramid* Activities

To bring alive the concepts of *MyPyramid*, plan activities that will engage students and make the food groups relevant to their lives.

ACTIVITY
▲ 16 USES FOR A BLANK PYRAMID

The blank *MyPyramid* on page 52 can be used in a variety of ways to teach *MyPyramid* concepts. Photocopy, enlarge or download the original from *http://teamnutrition.usda.gov/resources/mpk_coloring.pdf*. Assign children the following activities or create your own.

1. Display a colored poster or overhead of *MyPyramid for Kids*. (You can download one from *www.mypyramid.gov/kids*.) Pass out blank *MyPyramid* sheets and ask children to fill in the names of the food groups and color and label the bars.

> *Evaluation Tip: Upon completion of your nutrition unit, repeat this exercise without showing students the colored poster in advance.*

2. Bring in garden catalogs, food magazines and/or weekly food advertisements from the newspaper. Ask students to cut out the pictures and paste on the blank MyPyramid in the appropriate food group bands.

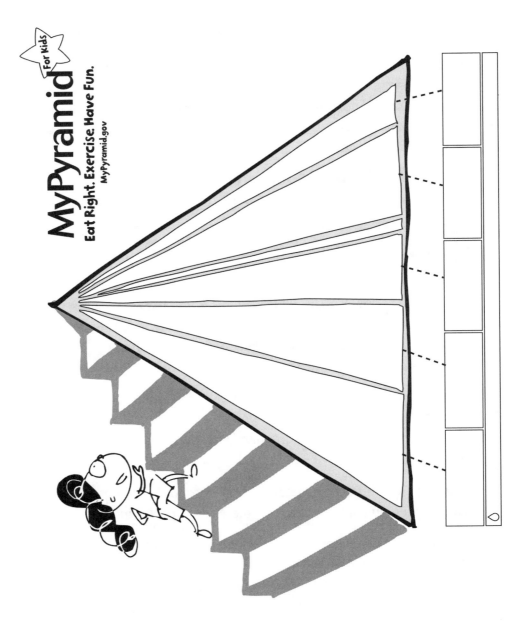

Source: Team Nutrition, USDA. Download a copy of this handout at *http://teamnutrition.usda.gov/resources/mpk_coloring.pdf*

3. Use the blank *MyPyramid* as a daily diet record. Carry it with you and record each food you eat or drink in the appropriate food group band. Break foods into their components (e.g., record a soup made of noodles, beef and vegetables in the grains, meat & bean, and vegetable groups). Check your record for balance. Is there a lot of blank space in certain groups? Are other groups overcrowded? Are there changes you could make to better balance *MyPyramid*?

4. Chart today's school breakfast or lunch menu on the *MyPyramid*. Are the menus balanced? Would you make any changes to the meals?

5. Ask the children who brought a packed lunch from home to analyze the contents and record them on the *MyPyramid*. Are most of the food groups represented? Would you make any changes to the meal?

6. Use the *MyPyramid* to plan your after-school or bedtime snack. Close your eyes and think about what foods are usually available in your refrigerator or cupboard. Next, think about which of these foods would make a good "*MyPyramid* snack." Write down or draw this snack on the blank *MyPyramid*. Be sure to include foods that you like to eat!

7. Plan a *MyPyramid* meal that you can cook yourself. It can be as simple as a peanut butter/fruit sandwich with milk or as complicated as a spaghetti dinner with salad. You're the cook!

8. Draw a vegetarian *MyPyramid*. What foods would you include in the meat & beans group? What about the milk group? Do vegetarians eat eggs? (ANSWER: Vegetarian diets are varied. Some, called lacto-vegetarians, include milk, yogurt and cheese in their diets. Lacto-ovo-vegetarians also eat eggs. Strict vegetarians, known as vegans, eat only plant-based foods and often include calcium-fortified soy milk and tofu in their diets.)

9. Draw an ethnic *MyPyramid*. Pick a culture that you are studying about or interested in and research what types of foods the members commonly eat. For example, a Mexican *MyPyramid* might include tortillas (grains), beans (meat & beans), cheese (milk) and salsa (vegetables). What would a Middle Eastern, Chinese or Italian *MyPyramid* look like?

10. Using the blank *MyPyramid*, dissect combination foods and write the components in the proper food group bands. Use one of the following examples or create your own:

> VEGETARIAN PIZZA: whole-wheat crust, tomato sauce with spices, part-skim mozzarella cheese, red pepper rings, mushrooms, onions, black olives

> CHINESE STIR-FRY: water chestnuts, bean sprouts, pea pods, broccoli florets, chicken pieces, peanuts, rice

> SUB SANDWICH: Whole-wheat hoagie roll, sliced turkey, lean ham, part-skim mozzarella cheese, tomato slices, shredded lettuce, pickle slices, oil, vinegar

11. Research the foods that are grown in your state or region. Design a "*MyPyramid* where I live," filling in all the agricultural products that you have identified in the correct food group spaces. A good resource for learning about agriculture in your state is *www.agclassroom.org*.

12. Research the nutrients that each food group provides. Write the key nutrients from each group on the blank *MyPyramid*. (ANSWERS: Grains — carbohydrate, fiber, B vitamins, iron; Vegetables — vitamins A and C, folate, iron, magnesium, fiber; Fruits — vitamins A and C, potassium, folate, fiber; Milk — calcium, vitamin D, riboflavin, potassium, protein; Meat & beans — protein, B vitamins, iron, zinc. Refer to Table 4-3 for more about specific nutrients.)

13. Draw a "body-part" *MyPyramid* that represents how each food group helps the body. EXAMPLE: Draw an exercising body in the grain space, healthy eyes in the vegetable group, glowing hair and skin for the fruit group, an arm posing a muscle in the meat & beans group and a healthy, toothy smile for the milk group.

14. Make a giant *MyPyramid* to decorate the school cafeteria. Start with a large blank *MyPyramid*. Assign seven students to the grains group, five to the vegetables group, three to the fruits group, three to the milk group, three to the meat & beans group (you may need to make adjustments according to class size). Have students design, draw, paint or color a favorite food from their assigned food group. Paste them on the large *MyPyramid* and hang it in the cafeteria. Be sure to have students sign their artwork.

Or, with the help of an artist or art teacher, have students design and paint a *MyPyramid* mural right on the cafeteria wall!

15. HOMEWORK: Accompany the "family shopper" on the next trip to the grocery store. Are most foods in the store from one of the five food groups? As the groceries are being put away at home, write down all the items on your blank *MyPyramid*. Is your *MyPyramid* balanced? What suggestions would you give the family shopper (nicely, of course!)?

16. Discuss why activity is now a part of *MyPyramid* (refer to chapter 11 for more on activity). Ask students to write their favorite physical activities on the steps of the blank *MyPyramid* sheet.

◼ MAKE A FOOD GROUP COUNTER

YOU WILL NEED:

For each Food Group Counter:

- shoebox
- string or twine
- 72 buttons or beads (evenly divided among six different colors)
- markers or crayons

Using a shoe box, string or twine and buttons or beads, children can make a device to help them count how many food group servings they eat each day. First, punch six small holes along one of the long sides of the shoe box. Punch six more on the other side that pair up with the first set of holes. Next, cut six pieces of string that are approximately twice the width of the box. Knot each piece of string and thread through the holes. Feed 12 beads or buttons onto each string. The last step is to thread the string through the opposite hole and tie a knot on the end to secure.

Each row of beads represents a food group. Match the bead/button colors to the groups if possible: grains:orange, vegetables:green, fruits:red, milk:blue, meat & beans:purple, and a separate color for "extras." NOTE: It is easier to write the food group names on the bottom of the box before stringing beads.

Ask students to write down the foods they eat each day. (The *MyPyramid* diet record suggested in #3 above works well.) Using their Food Group Counter, the students can move one bead to the opposite side for each serving they eat in that category. They can also do this for individual meals, snacks or school meal menus. This device will give students a visual tool that allows them to immediately gauge whether a meal or diet is balanced.

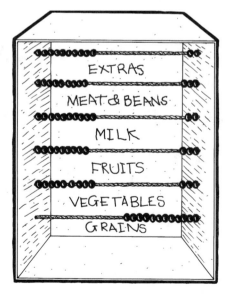

⊞ MEASURING CENTERS

Perhaps the biggest hang-up in applying the *MyPyramid* to daily eating habits is confusion over serving sizes (this is true of adults as well as children). Hands-on experience weighing and measuring different foods will give children a better grasp of what a "serving" really is.

Set up centers for children to manipulate and measure real food. Small food scales, measuring cups, measuring spoons, plates, cups and bowls are needed for this activity.

CAUTION: This is NOT an eating activity, since everyone will be touching the food. You may want to plan this activity in conjunction with a snack or conduct it right after lunch, when tummies are full!

Some suggestions for centers:

• Measure 1 ounce (1/2 cup) of cooked spaghetti, noodles, macaroni or rice onto a dinner-sized plate.

• Weigh 1-1/2 ounces of cheese in different forms, including sliced, cubed or grated.

• Measure one teaspoon of soft margarine or slice one "pat" of stick butter (using lines on butter wrapper).

• Pour 1 cup of 100 percent fruit juice into a glass.

• Using whole leaves from leaf lettuce or fresh spinach, tear into bite-sized pieces and measure 2 cups. How many lettuce leaves does it take to fill 2 cups?

• Weigh 1 ounce of drained, canned tuna fish.

YOU WILL NEED:

- Measuring cups
- Measuring spoons
- Food scale
- Serving utensils
- Plates, cups and bowls
- Cooked pasta or rice
- Cheese
- Butter or margarine
- Fruit juice
- Salad greens
- Tuna fish
- Items for "guess table" (see text)

• Set up a "guess table" with a variety of foods. The objective is to guess how many servings each food item really provides. Examples include an English muffin (2 ounces of grains), 1 cup canned fruit, 1 large orange (1 serving), 32 grapes, 1 cup cooked oatmeal (2 ounces grains), 1/2 pint carton of milk (1 cup), 1/2 ounce shelled sunflower seeds (1 ounce meat equivalent) or a 3-ounce cooked hamburger patty (3 ounces of meat).

🍽 Your school cafeteria manager is the real expert when it comes to serving sizes. Part of the manager's job is to serve the right-sized portions. Invite him/her into the classroom to demonstrate different scoops, scales and spoons used to control serving sizes. Also encourage students to take note of the serving sizes on their school breakfast and lunch trays. For instance, a typical pre-plated school lunch has 2 ounces of meat or protein, 1 cup of milk, 1–2 ounces of grains and (usually) 1/2 cup fruit and 1 cup of vegetable.

🐷 USING *MyPyramid* IN DRAMATIC PLAY AREAS

Setting up dramatic play areas is a great way for primary students (K-third grade) to play and practice the concepts of the *MyPyramid*.

▲ *MyPyramid* **Supermarket:** Set up a supermarket that is full of *MyPyramid* choices. Include shelves for food, grocery carts, aprons, cash register and grocery bags. Decorate the walls with student-made posters and advertisements.

YOU WILL NEED:

- Shelves
- A variety of empty food packages and/or food models
- Grocery carts
- Aprons
- Cash register
- Grocery sacks

For food models, use empty food packages (stuff items such as bread bags and flour sacks with pillow foam); canned goods; milk cartons; packages of rice, beans and pasta and plastic or rubber models of perishable items such as fruits, vegetables, meats and eggs. Include a wide variety of foods from all five food groups and a few foods from the "extras" category.

▲ *MyPyramid* **Kitchen:** Stock the dramatic play area kitchen with healthful *MyPyramid* choices. Include models of low-fat or fat-free milk, yogurt and cheese; lean meats, chicken and fish; whole grains, including 100 percent whole-wheat bread and flour and plenty of grains, beans, fruits and vegetables.

▲ **The** *MyPyramid* **Cafe:** Use glasses, plates, silverware, napkins and food pictures that students can make into meals. The food pictures can be preprinted, cut from magazines or food advertisements or made by students. Provide tables and chairs, student-created menus, aprons, chef hats, pads and pencils, a cash register and anything else your young restaurateurs need to run their cafe.

▲ *MyPyramid* **Felt Board:** Design a *MyPyramid* felt board in the shape of the *MyPyramid* with a variety of felt foods. (Encourage children to help you design and cut out the foods.) You can also feature a felt placemat with plate, dinnerware, glasses and napkins.

▲ **A** *MyPyramid* **PARTY:**
  CREATE YOUR OWN SANDWICH

A great cooking/tasting activity is to create *MyPyramid* sandwiches. Check with your cafeteria manager as a source for low-cost food supplies. If eaten as part of a reimbursable school meal, the food items will count as meal components. Funds for nutrition education projects may also be available from the local parent-teacher organization or through nutrition education grants.

> **YOU WILL NEED:**
>
> ■ Durable glasses, plates, silverware and napkins
>
> ■ Tables and chairs
>
> ■ Food models or sturdy food pictures
>
> ■ Aprons
>
> ■ Chef hats
>
> ■ Cash register
>
> ■ Pads and pencils
>
> ■ Menus (made by students)

NOTE: It is best to conduct this activity as part of lunch or at the end of the school day to avoid interfering with the school meal program.

- Plenty of volunteers!

- Variety of food items from each food group (see text for ideas)

- Serving utensils

- Long table

- Plastic or latex gloves

- Plates

- Plastic knives

- Napkins

Review Appendix A, "Guidelines for Safe Classroom Cooking," before setting up this activity. Be sure to enlist parent volunteers to help with this project.

To create *MyPyramid* sandwiches, make available a variety of items that can be combined in a large number of sandwich combinations. Try to have at least three choices from each food group available. Below are examples from each food category.

Grains: whole-wheat bread, rye bread, bagels, whole-wheat tortillas, English muffins, whole-wheat pita bread, hoagie rolls

Vegetables: lettuce or spinach leaves, tomato slices, cucumber slices, pepper rings, onion slices, mushroom slices, grated carrots, squash

Fruits: banana slices, raisins, applesauce, pineapple tidbits, blueberries, kiwifruit slices

Milk: low-fat ricotta cheese, low-fat cheese slices, low-fat grated cheese, fat-free plain and fruit-flavored yogurt

Meat & Beans: peanut butter; lean sliced turkey, ham or roast beef; water-packed tuna; refried beans

Extras: butter, margarine, mayonnaise, jam, jelly

Before you start, list all the available food items on the board. Explain that students will get a chance to build their own *MyPyramid* sandwich, using any combination of foods they wish. Encourage them to start thinking about the sandwich they wish to make — otherwise the line may move at a snail's pace! (An amusing book to read ahead of time is *What's Cooking, Jenny Archer?* by Ellen Conford — see page 77 for a detailed description.)

On a long table, set out items, grouped by food group. You will also need plastic gloves, plates, plastic knives for spreading and napkins. After thorough handwashing, let small groups of children come to the table. Instruct them to put on plastic gloves and refrain from touching their hair, face, clothing or neighbor.

Encourage students to experiment with new food combinations, building a sandwich that has at least three of the five food groups. After everyone has created a *MyPyramid* sandwich, it's time to eat the results!

FOLLOW-UP ACTIVITIES

Encourage students to write about their sandwich, including what they liked about it, how they would change it next time, how many food groups they used and whether they think their families or friends would eat it.

The food lists on the board can also be used

• to create additional sandwich combinations on paper that the children could try at home.

• to construct sentences or a story, using as many of the food words as possible.

• as weekly spelling words.

CHAPTER 5

Language Arts

"I really liked your lesson because we got to eat it." —Naveid

Children can discover a variety of nutrition concepts through language arts. Nutrition can be effectively integrated into reading, writing, storytelling and even spelling activities.

Daily Menu Reading

As you change the calendar and discuss the weather each day, consider another daily task — read and discuss the school lunch menu (and perhaps the following day's breakfast menu).

Assign a student to read the menu to the class. As time allows, ask students questions about the menu, such as:

▲ What food groups are represented in the menu? Does the menu fit the guidelines of *MyPyramid?* If there are a variety of food choices offered, is it easy to put together a breakfast or lunch that is nutritious and balanced? How many of the food choices would be classified as "extra" foods?

▲ Poll students to find out how many will eat the school meal. How many brought their lunch from home?

▲ Ask children what they like the most and least about the menu. Encourage them to fill in the blank, "If I were the cafeteria manager, I would serve _____."

Predict how many students school-wide will eat the school meal today. How can they find out the answer to their prediction? (HINT: Ask the cafeteria manager.)

Children's Books with Food Themes

Children's literature is full of books with whimsical food themes. Many of the titles below will stimulate discussion, serve as a prelude to a nutrition or cooking activity and promote positive food behavior.

EARLY ELEMENTARY (K–SECOND GRADES)

Bread and Jam for Frances, by Russell Hoban, HarperTrophy, 1993. This book is a perfect antidote for children who make limited food choices. Frances's food jag is short-lived once her parents begin serving her bread and jam for every meal and snack. In the end, she agrees with her friend Albert, who declares, "I think it's nice that there are all different kinds of lunches and breakfasts and dinners and snacks. I think eating is nice."

ACTIVITY

▲ Lead a discussion on how choosing a variety of different foods can make eating fun. Encourage children to draw pictures of two or more different breakfasts, lunches or dinners (with no repeating of foods) that they like to eat.

Blueberries for Sal, by Robert McCloskey, Puffin, 1976. Little Sal gets so involved picking (and eating) blueberries on Blueberry Hill that she loses her mother. Meanwhile, a baby bear cub does the same — and soon the baby bear and Little Sal have swapped moms!

ACTIVITIES

▲ Sample and rate a variety of berries, including blueberries, strawberries and raspberries.

▲ Research or discuss how blueberries and other berries grow.

▲ In late Spring/early Summer, take a field trip to a berry farm.

YOU WILL NEED:

- Different berries for tasting
- Serving bowls and utensils
- Small plates for tasting
- Clean hands
- Plastic gloves

Eating the Alphabet: Fruits & Vegetables from A to Z, by Lois Ehlert, Voyager Books, 1993. With beautiful watercolor illustrations, the art in this book will appeal to readers of all ages. The author includes well-known produce with the more exotic, including endive, jicama, kumquat, kohlrabi, quince, ugli fruit and xigua (Chinese watermelon). A highlight of the book is the glossary, which gives descriptions, origins and interesting facts about all of the fruits and vegetables in the book.

ACTIVITIES

▲ Bring in a variety of the fruits and vegetables from *Eating the Alphabet* to observe and taste.

▲ Take a walking field trip to a grocery market. Tour the produce section, noting the variety of produce available. Write about it later.

Encourage students to create and illustrate their own "*Eating the Alphabet*" books, using foods from any group they wish.

Assign each student a letter of the alphabet. Distribute brown paper bags and assorted art supplies, instructing students to make a puppet that represents a food of that letter. Use the puppets to create a skit or act out "The Alphabet Song" (see Chapter 9 for more ideas).

Eating Fractions, by Bruce McMillan, Scholastic Inc., 1991. A math book that whets the appetite, the bright color photos in this book show two kids eating delicious "fractions" of food. A banana, cloverleaf roll, vegetable pizza, corn on the cob, pear salad and strawberry pie illustrate math concepts. The author carries his

YOU WILL NEED:

- A variety of fruits and vegetables
- Cutting board and knife
- Serving bowls and utensils
- Small plates for tasting
- Clean hands
- Plastic gloves

YOU WILL NEED:

- Small paper lunch bags
- A variety of art supplies

math (and food) message one step further by including his recipes, which provide delicious practice learning fractions.

ACTIVITIES

▲ Use a cantaloupe or honeydew melon to illustrate fractions and provide a healthful snack. In a stepwise fashion, cut the melon in half, fourths, eighths, etc. depending on the size of the melon. Pass the pieces out for a snack, asking students what "fraction" of the whole they are eating.

▲ For homework, ask students to find and report on a "fraction" of a food they ate at home (e.g., 1/8 of a pizza, 1/12 of a casserole or 1/2 of an apple).

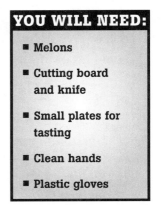

YOU WILL NEED:

- Melons
- Cutting board and knife
- Small plates for tasting
- Clean hands
- Plastic gloves

Fat, Fat Rose Marie, by Lisa Passen, Henry Holt, 1991. The new girl at school, Rose Marie endures cruel teasing by all of her classmates except Claire. Freckle-faced Claire notices Rose Marie's shiny blond hair, bright blue eyes and talent for math. Individual acceptance and the true meaning of friendship are themes explored in this book.

ACTIVITIES

▲ Lead a discussion on how people come in a variety of shapes, colors and sizes, pointing out that there is no one "best" way to look. Discuss the concept of prejudice and elicit ways that children can deal with mean teasing and cruel remarks.

Have students create life-sized self portraits, tracing their bodies onto large sheets of paper. Have them draw and color in the details, emphasizing their own unique qualities. Display them in the classroom or hallway.

Gobble and Gulp, by Stephen Cosgrove, Random House, 1985. One in a series of stories about the Whimsies, *Gobble and Gulp* tells of how the

Whimsies loved to grow and eat wholesome foods. But trouble brews for Whimsie twins Blossom and Sprout when they are placed under a spell from Switch Witch. They ignore the foods that are good for them and stuff themselves with sweets. The spell is broken when they discard the "Sweet Tooth" necklaces given to them by Switch Witch.

ACTIVITIES

▲ This book reinforces the role excessive sugar plays in tooth decay. Lead a discussion on how bacteria in the mouth love sugar, too! When the bacteria feed on sugars, acid is formed, which can harm teeth and result in cavities.

Conduct an experiment with soda pop and a tooth (ask your dentist for donations or use a baby tooth). Place the tooth in the soda pop and observe and record changes each day. The acid and sugar from the pop will eventually dissolve the tooth!

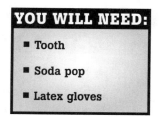

YOU WILL NEED:

- Tooth
- Soda pop
- Latex gloves

NOTE: When handling teeth, be sure to wear latex gloves to minimize the risk of disease transmission.

Good Morning, Little Fox, by Marilyn Janovitz, North-South Books, 2001. Father Fox doesn't think he likes porridge, so, naturally, Little Fox decides he doesn't care for it either. After their morning chores, they become so hungry that Little Fox convinces his father to try (and enjoy) the porridge!

ACTIVITIES

▲ Lead a discussion with the children about trying new foods. Ask questions such as: Have you ever decided whether you liked a food before you tasted it? Have you ever been surprised by the taste of a new food? Have you ever set a good example for others by trying new foods?

✖ Have students make their own "Good Morning" breakfast place mats out of construction paper, magazine pictures or their own art that illustrates the importance of a healthful breakfast.

Green Eggs and Ham, by Dr. Seuss, Random House, 1960. Tongue-tied teachers and parents can take refuge in the fact that *Green Eggs and Ham* does make an important point about food — you will never know if you like a new food until you try it. That now-classic refrain is as pertinent today as ever: "You do not like them. So you say. Try them! Try them! And you may. Try them and you may, I say."

ACTIVITY

▲ Have children think of foods that they are hesitant to try, either at home or at school. Award "Sam-I-Am" points each time children try any new food of their choice. Reward students with small incentives or privileges after they attain a certain number of points.

Gregory the Terrible Eater, by Mitchell Sharmat, Scholastic, 1989. A classic tale about the struggles parents and "kids" have over food choices. Gregory the goat refuses the usual goat fare of shoes, old neckties and tin cans in favor of fruits, vegetables, eggs and orange juice.

ACTIVITY

▲ There are a lot of different foods from which to choose. Ask children whether it is OK to like some foods better than others.

▲ Point out that this is a silly, funny story. While goats do sometimes nibble on paper and clothing, those are not the foods real goats subsist on. Ask children if they have ideas about what goats really do eat. (ANSWER: hay, alfalfa, oats, corn and apples.)

Encourage students to design finger and stick puppets of food and other characters and perform a puppet show (Gregory the goat might be one of the characters).

I Will Never Not Ever Eat a Tomato, by Lauren Child, Candlewick Press, 2000. Lola is a fussy eater until her big brother Charlie makes up inventive names for vegetables and other foods. Carrots become "orange twiglets from Jupiter," peas are "green drops from Greenland" and mashed potatoes turn into "cloud fluff from the pointiest peak of Mount Fuji."

ACTIVITY

▲ Ask children to list their ten favorite foods. Next, ask them to make up inventive names for the foods and use the words to write their own creative story.

Junie B. Jones, First Grader: Boss of Lunch, by Barbara Park, Random House, 2002. In this Junie B. adventure, she is making trouble in the cafeteria. This hilarious book is supportive of the school meal program and sheds a positive light on "cafeteria ladies."

ACTIVITY

▲ Invite the cafeteria manager or food service director to the classroom to discuss how the school lunch menus are designed to meet the nutritional needs of students. End the lesson by taking a field trip to the school kitchen.

Mrs. Pig's Bulk Buy, by Mary Rayner, Atheneum, 1990. This book provides yet another twist on the theme that variety is essential when making food choices. Mrs. Pig teaches her ten piglets a lesson when they insist on dumping ketchup on everything, even toast, salad and eggs! On her next trip to the store, she buys six enormous jars of ketchup. At first, the piglets are excited that they get so much of their favorite food. But once they realize that's all they get, they soon crave real food. The fanciful illustrations in this book show the little pigs gradually changing from white to pink.

ACTIVITY

▲ Set up the following scenario for children: If you could eat only one food, what would it be? How soon would you get tired of this food? Write a make-believe story of what might happen if you ate too much of this one food.

Oliver's Milkshake, by Vivian French, Orchard Books, 2001. In this story, Oliver visits a dairy farm with his aunt and cousin. They make a delicious milkshake from fresh milk, blueberries, a banana and ice.

ACTIVITY

▲ Try the following fruit smoothie recipe:

So-Berry-Good Smoothies

Ingredients:
1 cup frozen berries (strawberries, blueberries or raspberries)
1 frozen banana, broken into chunks
1 cup vanilla yogurt
1 cup fat-free or 1% milk
2–4 tsp. sugar (depending on the sweetness of the berries)

YOU WILL NEED:
- Ingredients for smoothie recipe (see text)
- Blender
- Small cups or glasses for tasting

Combine all ingredients in the blender; process until smooth. Serve immediately. Makes 4 servings.

Rabbit Food, by Susanna Gretz, Candlewick Press, 1999. John is a young rabbit who doesn't like vegetables ("rabbit food"). Uncle Bunny comes to the rescue, except he tries to hide the fact that he doesn't like carrots!

ACTIVITY

▲ For a homework assignment, ask children to think up a new way to eat carrots ("rabbit food"). Ideas include using grated carrots in pancakes, pasta sauce, salads or soup, serving carrot sticks dipped in peanut butter or sprinkling raisins on cooked carrots. Encourage them to try their ideas out on their families and write down the recipes.

Stone Soup, by Marcia Brown, Scott Foresman, 1997. A classic story of how three hungry soldiers convince the peasants of a small village that soup made of stones is indeed hearty and delicious. As the soldiers begin heating up their soup of water and three polished stones, the peasants eagerly contribute ingredients, including a few carrots, some cabbage, a little barley, beef, potatoes and milk, until finally the soldiers declare the soup "fit for a King."

ACTIVITY

▲ As a class, create a pot of vegetable-stone soup, using a crock pot and clean stone. Use tomato or vegetable juice for the base, add salt, pepper, and desired seasonings, and ask each child to bring a fresh vegetable from home. Assemble first thing in the morning, cook on high and eat for a snack during the later part of the school day!

The Berenstain Bears and Too Much Junk Food, by Stan and Jan Berenstain, Random House, 1985. When Mama Bear notices her two cubs getting a little chubby, she decides to curtail their junk-food habits. To his surprise, Papa Bear must forgo much of his junk food as well. Great family reading, the Berenstains do an excellent job of covering basic nutrition principles, the importance of a healthy lifestyle and the role exercise plays in good health.

YOU WILL NEED:

- Crock pot
- Clean stone
- Tomato or vegetable juice
- Salt, pepper, seasonings
- Assorted vegetables (from children's homes)
- Soup ladle
- Bowls and spoons
- Clean hands
- Plastic gloves

ACTIVITIES

▲ Ask each child to write down or draw pictures of physical activities that his or her family can do together.

▲ Lead a discussion on how exercise and nutrition work together to produce fit young bodies.

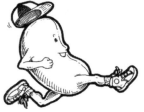

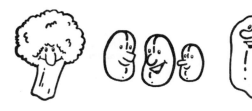

The Hatseller and the Monkeys, by Baba Wagué Diakité, Scholastic, 1999. In this authentic African tale, hatseller BaMusa forgets to eat breakfast before he takes off on a day-long journey. He soon falls asleep under a mango tree and the monkeys make off with his hats. Only after he eats is he able to think clearly and devise a way to get his hats back.

ACTIVITIES

▲ Have students write a story or draw a picture about the importance of breakfast and how it "wakes up the brain" and helps them to think and learn.

▲ Hold a mango tasting. Demonstrate how to peel and slice a fresh mango, show children the long oblong seed and pass out samples to taste.

YOU WILL NEED:

- Mangoes
- Sharp knife
- Small plates for tasting
- Clean hands
- Plastic gloves

The Little Red Hen (authors, publishers, and versions vary slightly — I prefer the version where she makes bread, not cake). While this classic sends a strong message about work, cooperation and consequences, an underlying theme teaches children the stages of bread production. From wheat seed to bread, the Little Red Hen perseveres in her production of a loaf of bread.

ACTIVITIES

▲ Use visual props and a baking activity to tell the story. Obtain wheat kernels (purchase from mills or specialty grocery stores), stalks of dried wheat (available in craft stores), whole-wheat flour and whole-wheat bread dough (from scratch or purchased frozen). After the story, divide the bread dough into roll-sized portions for each student. Encourage children to create their own "bread art" by kneading and shaping the dough. Line the baking tray with parchment baking paper, label each child's bread art, bake according to package or recipe instructions and serve as a snack. (You may want to enlist the help of your cafeteria manager with this project.)

▪ Using potting soil and small containers (empty milk cartons work great), have students plant the wheat kernels and care for their plants. (See Chapter 7 for more on growing plants.)

YOU WILL NEED:

- Wheat kernels
- Dried wheat stalks
- Whole-wheat flour
- Whole-wheat bread dough
- Clean work surface
- Parchment baking paper
- Baking trays
- Oven
- Napkins or small plates
- Clean hands
- Plastic gloves

The Little Red Hen (Makes a Pizza!), by Philemon Sturges, Dutton Children's Books, 1999. The industrious Little Red Hen is back with a modern spin! This whimsical and updated version is entertaining and also a good excuse to make a pizza from scratch.

ACTIVITY

▲ Try the "perfectly personal pizza" recipe on page 98.

The Very Hungry Caterpillar, by Eric Carle, Scholastic, 1994. This story clearly and vividly illustrates how food is needed to build young bodies. The caterpillar, with his insatiable appetite, eventually grows big and prepares to turn into a beautiful butterfly. This book sets the stage for a discussion of how food fuels the growth of all living things, even kids.

ACTIVITIES

▲ Encourage children to create a story about "The Very Hungry Kid," complete with the foods they (or the character they create) would choose to eat on each day of the week and the resultant growth that occurs.

▲ To measure how food fuels the growth of children, start a classroom growth chart. Take measurements each month, noting the changes as the year progresses.

Nonfiction Nutrition Books for Early Elementary

The following nutrition books teach and reinforce basic nutrition principles and can be used as reference books for students.

Good Enough to Eat: A Kid's Guide to Food and Nutrition, by Lizzy Rockwell, HarperCollins, 1999.

Gobble Up Science, by Carol A. Johmann and Elizabeth Rieth, Learning Works, 1996.

Gobble Up Math, by Sue Mogard and Ginny McDonnell, Learning Works, 1994.

UPPER ELEMENTARY (THIRD–FIFTH GRADES)

Annie Pitts, Artichoke, by Diane deGroat, SeaStar Books, 2001. Third-grader Annie Pitts is determined to become a famous actress. But she fails to get the lead in the class nutrition play after a food fight with Matthew at the supermarket field trip. Forced to play the artichoke (and a last minute fill-in for the fish), Annie manages to put on a performance that nobody will forget! Students will enjoy this humorous book as they learn a few nutrition concepts, too.

ACTIVITY

As a class or in small groups, stage a nutrition play. See Chapter 9 for ideas.

Nothing's Fair in Fifth Grade, by Barthe DeClements, Puffin, 1990. Written by a school counselor, this fictional story explores the psychological issues surrounding childhood obesity. Not only is Elsie Edwards the new girl at school, she is also obese and considered "gross" by classmates. Elsie's classmates eventually accept her and she begins to lose weight. This book teaches valuable lessons about the prejudice and cruelty endured by overweight people in our society.

ACTIVITY

▲ Lead a discussion on how people come in a variety of shapes and sizes, pointing out that there is no one "best" way to look.

Pig and the Shrink, by Pamela Todd, Delacorte Press, 1999. Tucker learns about life, friendship and ambition when he decides to use fat kid "Pig" (Angelo Pighetti) as his science project. Tucker's efforts at changing Pig's eating habits backfire, Pig gains even more weight during the experiment and Tucker fears he has lost a good friend. This humorous book sends a strong message about acceptance.

ACTIVITY

▲ Discuss with students the ethics of changing people because *you* want them to change. Ask whether they think it is acceptable to tell another person what to eat. Ask whether they want someone else to control *their* eating or exercise habits.

Is there a way to help people without forcing them to change? Ask students to note the difference between helping a friend and hurting a friend. Suggest they write papers on how they would help friends with nutrition or weight problems.

What's Cooking, Jenny Archer?, by Ellen Conford, Little, Brown, and Co., 1991. A "creative" cook who enjoys sandwiches made with mint jelly and bologna on raisin bread, Jenny begins concocting her own lunches for school. Soon her friends want her to make their lunches, too. Figuring she will quickly get rich, Jenny sets out to sell creative lunches to her friends. Her plan backfires when she is unable to please the picky palates of her friends.

ACTIVITIES

▲ Create an original "*MyPyramid* sandwich." (See page 60.)

🍴 Invite the school nutrition manager to class to discuss how he or she manages to meet the tastes and preferences of all the children in the school. Suggest that the class assist the manager in planning a school breakfast or lunch menu.

Nonfiction Food & Nutrition Books for Upper Elementary

The following books convey basic nutrition principles, serve as reference books and feature recipes and experiments that teach and reinforce food and nutrition concepts.

The Healthy Body Cookbook: Over 50 Fun Activities and Delicious Recipes for Kids, by Joan D'Amico and Karen Eich Drummond, John Wiley, 1999.

The Science Chef Travels Around the World: Fun Food Experiments and Recipes for Kids, by Joan D'Amico and Karen Eich Drummond, John Wiley, 1996.

Janice Vancleave's Food and Nutrition for Every Kid: Easy Activities That Make Learning Science Fun, by Janice Pratt Vancleave, John Wiley, 1999.

The Kids' Multicultural Cookbook: Food & Fun Around the World, by Deanna F. Cook, Williamson Publishing, 1995.

Food Rules! The Stuff You Munch, Its Crunch, Its Punch, and Why You Sometimes Lose Your Lunch, by Bill Haduch and Rick Stromoski (Illustrator), 2001.

Putting a Nutrition Twist on Fairy Tales

Once upon a time, there was an enchanted school cafeteria where the princess ate her peas, the porridge was always "just right," a vegetarian wolf never bothered the three little pigs and the breakfast eggs were laid by a prized golden goose.

A fun activity that sharpens writing, illustrating, storytelling and comprehension skills is to retell classic stories, adding a nutritional bent. The possibilities for student assignments are endless. Below are a few examples.

ACTIVITIES

▲ Remember Jack Sprat who ate no fat and his wife who ate no lean? What would you tell Jack and Mrs. Sprat about nutritional moderation?

▲ Write a letter to "Baby Bear," giving him ideas on added ingredients that would make his porridge extra delicious and nutritious.

▲ If Little Red Riding Hood were really concerned about her sick grandmother's health, what "goodies" should she pack in the basket that would help Granny recover and stay healthy?

▲ Imagine that the witch in "Hansel and Gretel" was really a good witch, concerned with the nutritional health of the children who came to visit. Instead of gingerbread and candy, of what foods would her house be made?

▲ In the story of the grasshopper and the ant, the ant stocked up for the winter while the grasshopper failed to plan and went hungry. What advice would you give the grasshopper on collecting and storing food for the winter?

▲ The story of "Jack and the Beanstalk" fails to tell about the crop of beans that must have resulted from such a large plant. Write or tell about what Jack and his mom did with all those beans. Were they green beans or dried beans? Did they eat them or sell them? How did they cook them? Any recipe ideas?

▲ When Winnie-the-Pooh indulges himself with too much honey and condensed milk at Rabbit's house, he gets stuck attempting to exit Rabbit's hole! How could Pooh Bear improve his eating and exercise habits so he doesn't get stuck the next time?

▲ Ask students to develop storybook names for menu items served during the month. Examples include Peter Piper's Pepper Pizza, Jack Sprat's No-Fat Ranch Dressing, Three Bear Breakfast Porridge Bar (with hot and cold cereals), Little Miss Muffet's Muffins (good served with curds and whey, or milk/yogurt if you insist), Jack Horner's Fresh Plums (sans thumb, thank you) or Jack-and-the-Beanstalk's green beans.

Children's tales with a reference to food or eating

Traditional Stories:
   Goldilocks and the Three Bears
   Jack and the Beanstalk
   Little Red Riding Hood
   The Little Gingerbread Man

Aesop's Fables:
   The Ant and the Grasshopper
   The Fox and the Grapes
   The Town Mouse and the Country Mouse
   The Goose with the Golden Eggs

Grimm's Fairy Tales
   Cinderella
   Hansel and Gretel
   Snow White

Mother Goose's Nursery Rhymes
   The Old Woman Who Lived in a Shoe
   Hey Diddle, Diddle
   Old Mother Hubbard
   Sing a Song of Sixpence
   Peter Piper
   Jack Sprat
   Little Miss Muffet
   This Little Pig Went to Market

American Tales
   Johnny Appleseed
   Paul Bunyan

Descriptive Writing

Using food as a subject is an effective way to develop descriptive writing skills. While children may have limited experience in other areas, they encounter food several times each day. The novice writer can more easily describe scenes and objects that are based on firsthand experience. Some ideas include:

ACTIVITIES

▲ The sight, smell and taste of food can evoke strong emotions. Suggest that students write about a particular meal or food that made them feel especially happy, excited, sentimental, sad, grouchy or even angry. Encourage them to provide details regarding the surroundings, people, food and why they felt as they did.

▲ Bring in colorful pictures, posters or samples of real food. Assign students the task of describing one food, using as many details as possible.

▲ Bring in various foods for a snack or tasting. Ask students to write down how different foods appeal to each of their five senses. For example, "The strawberry is a beautiful, red color with seeds that remind me of polka dots." "When I bite into a carrot, the crunchy sound fills up my whole head." "The smell of fresh bread makes me feel warm and happy clear down to my toes."

YOU WILL NEED:

- Colorful food pictures

OR

- A variety of real food samples to observe, smell and taste

Writing Activities for the Young Nutrition Advocate

Starting at a young age, it is important that kids learn to voice their opinions about policies and messages that affect their nutrition choices. The goal of writing letters should be to communicate opinions in a clear, constructive manner. Two areas to target include school meals and food advertisements.

SCHOOL MEALS

ACTIVITIES

▲ Begin by writing letters to the school nutrition manager or district nutrition director. Suggest that children begin the letter by stating what they like best about the school meals. If there are comments, suggestions or criticisms, word them in a constructive way (e.g., "One change I would like to see in the menu/cafeteria is _____" or "My idea of the perfect school breakfast/lunch menu is _____.").

▲ Write or send an e-mail to the United States Department of Agriculture (USDA), the federal agency that oversees child nutrition programs, including school breakfast, lunch and summer feeding programs. Communicate what you like the best about the school meal program and changes that you would like to see implemented. Address your letters to: Department of Agriculture, Office of The Secretary, 14th and Independence Ave SW, Room 200A, Washington, DC 20250; E-mail: *agsec@usda.gov*

FOOD ADVERTISEMENTS

ACTIVITIES

▲ The next time you are watching television on Saturday morning, keep a list of the advertised foods that are low in nutrition such as candy, pop or sugary cereal. Also keep a list of ads for healthful foods from the five food groups. Are there more ads for healthful foods or low-nutrition foods? (See worksheet on page 145.) You can write letters to those responsible for the ads, including the food company who advertises or the network itself.

To find the address for the food company, look at the food package the next time you go to the grocery store (or ask an adult to do it for you). Printed on the package is an address or e-mail that you can write to to voice your opinion.

▲ Write or send an e-mail to the television networks and let them know how you feel about their food advertising. The major networks can be reached at the following addresses:

- ABC, Inc., 77 West 66th Street, 3rd Floor, New York, NY 10023

- CBS Television Network, 51 West 52nd Street, New York, NY 10019, (212) 975-4321

- NBC, 30 Rockefeller Plaza, New York, NY 10112

- Nickelodeon, 1515 Broadway, 20th Floor, New York, NY 10036

- FOX Broadcasting, 10201 West Pico Boulevard, Los Angeles, CA 90035

You can also file a complaint by contacting the Children's Advertising Review Unit, a division of the Better Business Bureau at the following address:

Children's Advertising Review Unit, 70 West 36th Street, 13th Floor, New York, NY 10018, (866) 334-6272 (ext. 111)

SPELLING LIST

Include food, nutrition and fitness words in your list of weekly spelling words. Examples are listed below.

Aerobic	Fitness	Protein
Carbohydrate	Flexibility	Strength
Dairy	Fruit	Vegetable
Diet	Grain	Vitamin
Dietitian	Healthy	Water
Exercise	Mineral	Weight
Fat	Nutrient	
Fiber	Nutrition	

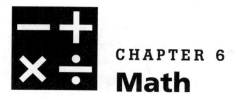

CHAPTER 6
Math

"I liked it when you showed us how much fat and sugar were in those two lunches. I was surprised when you showed us how much fat was in the lunch with the Big Mac. I thought that was kind of gross." —Dawn

The subjects of Nutrition and Math are easily integrated and mutually beneficial. Whether counting daily servings from the food groups, calculating nutrients or learning how to decipher the *Nutrition Facts* food label, the application of nutrition requires basic math skills. Likewise, math skills can be learned or reinforced through the use of real-life food activities by working with a recipe, dividing up portions or making purchases at the food market.

One food-related math skill that comes naturally to children, even the very young, is division. Children think of it as "fair share," always mindful that they get their deserved allotment of animal crackers, grapes or apple wedges. Build this natural inclination into a snacktime math lesson, using examples such as "There are 25 crackers left for table A — since there are five of you, how many do you each get?" Conversely, ask children how many graham crackers you need to buy if each student typically eats three squares.

Teaching Label Lessons

Label reading helps children sharpen their nutrition, math and critical thinking skills. The following activities will help children interpret and apply the *Nutrition Facts* label information.

Table 6-1

LEARNING TO USE
THE *NUTRITION FACTS* FOOD LABEL

The *Nutrition Facts* food label makes it easy for kids to decipher the sugar content of fruit drinks, compare the fat in different types of deli meat or check the fiber in various brands of breakfast cereal. Labeling laws require a *Nutrition Facts* label on all packaged foods and fresh meats. Nutrition information is also available in the produce and seafood sections for the 20 most commonly eaten raw fruits/vegetables and seafood.

The following points will help you to decipher the information found on food labels:

- The first thing to look at on a label is the serving size and number of servings per container. What appears to be a "single-serving" container can often contain two to three servings.

- Labels generally contain four key nutrients of special concern: vitamin A, vitamin C, calcium and iron. This doesn't mean that there are not other vitamins, minerals and phytochemicals in the food. Generally, though, if a food is high in these four key nutrients, it likely contains other important nutrients. Manufacturers may include information on additional nutrients on a voluntary basis.

- Labels include values for sugar and dietary fiber. Once optional on the label, sugars, starches and fiber were often lumped together under the carbohydrates heading. This information is especially handy when making comparisons of kids' favorite breakfast cereals.

- The *Nutrition Facts* label makes it easy to calculate the percentage of calories from fat in a food product. (See Table 6-2 for calculation). Keep in mind, though, that the goal to slide under 30 percent calories from fat applies to the diet as a whole, not to individual foods. Even a high-fat hunk of cheese can be tempered by pairing it with low-fat crackers and fruit wedges.

- Daily values (DV) show the contribution that each targeted nutrient makes to the daily diet. Expressed as a percentage, the DV tells you whether a food is high or low in a nutrient such as fat, sodium, cholesterol or vitamin C. In general, a food with a %DV of 5 percent or less for a nutrient is considered low in that nutrient, a product is considered a "good source" of a nutrient if the %DV is 10–19 percent and "high" if the %DV is greater than 20 percent.

Table 6-1 (continued)

- *Nutrition Facts* labels feature a standard chart that targets the daily recommended levels for fats, cholesterol, sodium, carbohydrate and fiber at 2,000 and 2,500 calories. While a child's nutrient needs are highly individual, these reference values give a "ballpark" goal for daily intake. Estimated caloric needs of children range from 1,800 for the average 4- to 6-year-old to 2,000 for a typical 7- to 10-year-old.
- Food labels require complete ingredient lists, even for those foods that use the government's "standard" recipes, such as mayonnaise, ketchup or jelly. This feature is especially important for those who have allergies or sensitivities to specific food additives.
- For more information and updates on *Nutrition Facts* food labels, visit the government food labeling and nutrition Web site at *vm.cfsan.fda.gov/label.html*

ACTIVITIES

▲ WHAT'S YOUR SERVING SIZE?

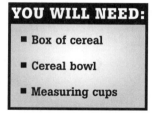

YOU WILL NEED:

- Box of cereal
- Cereal bowl
- Measuring cups

The "serving size" listed on a product label is often different from what we think of as a "helping." To make this point, bring in a large box of breakfast cereal, cereal bowls and measuring cups. Cover or remove the *Nutrition Facts* label information from the box. Ask children, a few at a time, to pour themselves a "bowl of cereal," typical of what they would eat for breakfast or a snack. Next, have students measure and record how much they poured into the bowl. After everyone has taken a turn, appoint one child to read aloud the serving amount listed on the label. Ask how many children measured the same amount, more or less than the label serving size. Remind students that the nutrition information on the remainder of the label pertains to the standard label serving size. Ask what that means in different situations (e.g., "If a label lists 4 grams of dietary fiber and your serving size is half as much as the standard serving, how many grams of fiber did you eat?").

Nutrition Facts

Serving Size ½ cup (114g)
Servings Per Container 4

Amount Per Serving

Calories 90   Calories from Fat 30

	% Daily Value*
Total Fat 3g	**5%**
Saturated Fat 0g	**0%**
Cholesterol 0mg	**0%**
Sodium 300mg	**13%**
Total Carbohydrate 13g	**4%**
Dietary Fiber 3g	**12%**
Sugars 3g	
Protein 3g	

Vitamin A	80%	Vitamin C	60%
Calcium	4%	Iron	4%

* Percent Daily Values are based on a 2,000 calorie diet. Your daily values may be higher or lower depending on your calorie needs:

	Calories	2,000	2,500
Total Fat	Less than	65g	80g
Sat Fat	Less than	20g	25g
Cholesterol	Less than	300mg	300mg
Sodium	Less than	2,400mg	2,400mg
Total Carbohydrate		300g	375g
Fiber		25g	30g

Calories per gram:
Fat 9 • Carbohydrate 4 • Protein 4

Source: Food & Drug Administration

OPTIONAL: Make a class graph that visually shows individual differences in serving sizes. Have each student plot his or her serving amount on a poster-sized bar graph. Include a comparison bar that shows the serving size listed on the label.

▲ CALORIES FROM FAT

Calories in food come from either carbohydrate, protein or fat. When gauging the nutritional merit of a food item, it is often helpful to look at the number of calories that come from fat. That is why "Calories from Fat" is listed next to "Calories" on the *Nutrition Facts* label.

Over the course of a day, the recommended goal is to eat a maximum of 30 percent of calories from fat. That does not mean every single food must fall below the 30 percent goal — higher-fat foods can be balanced with lower-fat foods to obtain a daily average of around 30 percent.

To obtain calories from fat in a given food, simply divide "Calories from Fat" by "Total Calories," and multiply by 100 for the percentage. This exercise is especially helpful when comparing two similar food items. (See Table 6-2.)

Using the *Nutrition Facts* label, encourage students to calculate the percentage of calories from fat in several food products.

What about "trans fat"?

Trans fatty acids are formed when food manufacturers hydrogenate vegetable oil to make it more solid. Trans fats are found in foods containing "hydrogenated" or "partially hydrogenated" vegetable oils. Examples include certain margarines, baked goods, snack foods and many other processed foods.

Trans fats have been shown to raise blood cholesterol levels and contribute to the development of heart disease. Most nutrition experts recommend limiting the intake of trans fat as much as possible. Beginning in 2006, food manufacturers are required to list the amount of trans fat on every food that carries a *Nutrition Facts* label.

NOTE: Since students don't always have access to calculators, pencils or paper, encourage the use of estimation in evaluating the nutrition content of foods. For example, the estimated fat content of a package of cookies with 65 calories per serving and 35 calories from fat would be "slightly more than one-half of the calories."

Table 6-2

HOW TO CALCULATE PERCENT CALORIES FROM FAT

To calculate percent calories from fat using the *Nutrition Facts* food label, you need the TOTAL CALORIES and CALORIES FROM FAT. Simply divide CALORIES FROM FAT by TOTAL CALORIES and multiply by 100 to arrive at the percentage.
The equation looks like this:

$$\frac{\text{Calories from Fat}}{\text{Total Calories}} \times 100 = \% \text{ Calories from Fat}$$

Example: A box of snack crackers provides 70 calories for a serving of 5 crackers. The "calories from fat" are listed as 20.

$$\frac{20}{70} \times 100 = 28.6\% \text{ Calories from Fat}$$

▲ MAKING COMPARISONS

The food label is a powerful tool for comparing similar food products. Younger children can begin by comparing one nutrient in different products, while students in the intermediate grades can learn to compare several parameters on a label. Suggest that students develop graphs or pictures with fractional pieces to illustrate the differences between foods.

Ten suggestions for comparing labels, ranked from simple to more complex, are listed below.

1. Sugar in Breakfast Cereal: Bring in a variety of cereal boxes. Locate "Sugars" on the label. On a piece of paper, rank the cereals in order of sugar content.

2. Total Fat in Crackers: Rank various crackers in order of "total fat" content.

3. Fat in Snack Foods: Compare the fat content in one serving of pretzels, chips, packaged popcorn and snack crackers.

4. Fiber in Bread: Just because a bread is dark in color, does not mean it's necessarily full of fiber. Compare the "Dietary Fiber" content of white bread, 100 percent whole-wheat bread and bread that is simply labeled "wheat."

5. Sugars in Unlikely Places: Various forms of sugar are commonly added to foods, even those we don't think of as "sweet." Send children on a "scavenger hunt" for foods that contain added sugars, such as ketchup, spaghetti sauce, mayonnaise, baked beans, hot dogs and certain breads.

6. Rating Lunch Meats: There is a notable difference in the fat, calorie and sodium content of luncheon meats. For homework or as part of a class field trip, assign students the task of finding and comparing at least five different lunch meats (e.g., lean ham or roast beef, different types of turkey meat, bologna and salami). Note the difference in calories, fat and sodium for a standard serving size. Which products are the best overall choices?

7. The Merits of Milk: "Two percent" milk sounds like it must be low in fat, but is it? Write down the Total Fat, Calories and Calories from Fat for fat-free, 1 percent, 2 percent and whole milk. Have students calculate the "percent calories from fat" in all four milks. Ask students why milk listed as 1 percent or 2 percent fat appears much higher in fat when using the "percent calories from fat" calculation. (ANSWER: 1 percent or 2 percent refers to fat by weight, which is low since most of the weight in milk comes from water.)

OPTIONAL: Compare the calcium content among different varieties of milk.

OPTIONAL: Compare the fat, sugar and calorie content of various frozen desserts, including ice cream, ice milk, frozen yogurt and sherbet.

8. Finding the "Better Butter": Although spreads such as butter, butter blends and margarines are, by nature, mostly fat, the key nutritional difference is the amount of fat that derives from either trans fat or saturated fat. (Both trans fats and saturated fats are associated with higher blood cholesterol and an increased risk for heart disease in later life.)

Ask children to look at a variety of labels and rank them by the level of trans and saturated fats. Note that there is a large difference in the saturated fat content of liquid, soft tub and stick margarines. Students will discover that certain margarines have nearly as much saturated fat as butter!

Keep in mind, too, that the flavor of butter is preferred by many, especially chefs and those involved in fine food preparation. Their advice: Use real butter — just use less of it!

9. Noodle Know-How: Kids may be surprised to learn that many brands of ramen noodles fare worse in fat and sodium content than an average serving of potato chips! Encourage students to read and evaluate their favorite ramen noodle labels. Ask them to look for brands that are lower in fat during their next trip to the grocery store.

OPTIONAL: Ask students how the nutrition of ramen noodles compares to standard egg noodles.

10. Taking a Closer Look at Fruit(?) Snacks: If you believe the advertising and packaging, there are a whole array of processed "fruit snacks" just loaded with fruit. To dispel this myth, teach students how to read ingredient labels on packaged foods, pointing out that ingredients are listed from most to least, by weight. Ask them to read the ingredient labels on a variety of fruit snacks to see in what order "fruit" or "fruit juice concentrate" falls in the ingredient list. Usually the "fruit" is listed third or fourth, behind various types of sugar, corn syrup and gelatin.

Measuring Nutrients in Food

Children can best grasp the concept of "high fat" or "high sugar" when they can actually see the fat and sugar in a food. The activities below give students practice in weighing and measuring, provide reference for what a "gram" is and visually display the fat and sugar content of various foods.

ACTIVITIES

▲ WHAT'S A GRAM?

Nutrient information on food labels, recipes, restaurant brochures and reference tables is mostly metric, with food components measured in grams and milligrams (1/1000 of a gram). Some nutrients, such as vitamin D and iodine, are needed in such small amounts that they are measured in micrograms (one millionth of a gram!).

The weight of a gram is approximately that of a small paper clip. Using a gram scale, ask students to weigh different common items such as a paper clip, pencil, eraser or chalk.

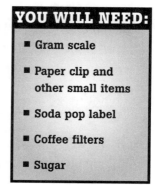

YOU WILL NEED:

- Gram scale
- Paper clip and other small items
- Soda pop label
- Coffee filters
- Sugar

Next, explain how the weights of many of the nutrients in foods are also listed in grams. The average 12-ounce can of soda pop, for instance, contains about 40 grams of sugar. To demonstrate, first place a coffee filter on top of the scale. Next, show the students how to "zero" the scale. Fill the coffee filter with sugar until the scale registers 40 grams, resulting in a small mountain of sugar!

▲ SETTING UP A CENTER

To set up a center for students to weigh and measure the fat and sugar in foods, you will need a gram scale, teaspoons, one pound of sugar, one pound of vegetable shortening, coffee filters, small plastic plates and food packages or labels.

Another way to measure grams is to use a teaspoon. A teaspoon of sugar or fat weighs approximately 4 grams, so students can measure the teaspoons of fat and sugar in food by dividing the total grams by 4.

On a long table, set out a variety of food packages or labels. Examples include candy bars, granola bars, yogurt containers, cereal boxes, potato chips, pretzels, crackers, cookies and fast food containers (nutrient information, including fat and sugar content, is usually available in the restaurant or at the restaurant's Web site).

A few at a time, students will read the labels and measure the fat and sugar content of the different food items, using coffee filters for sugar and plastic plates for fat. Have them place the containers with fat and sugar in front of each food package or label until they have measured all foods. When they are done, instruct them to scoop the fat and sugar back into the original containers and allow another group of students to work the center. (NOTE: Plastic plates can be washed and reused many times.)

OPTIONAL: Consider a semipermanent display of the fat and sugar in foods for the classroom or cafeteria. Invite other classes to observe and comment.

OPTIONAL: Using food labels, measure the fiber content (in grams) in a variety of breads and cereals, using bran cereal to represent fiber.

YOU WILL NEED:

- Gram scale
- Teaspoons
- One pound of sugar
- One pound of vegetable shortening
- Coffee filters
- Small plastic plates
- Food packages or labels

Graphing

A visual way to present and evaluate information is through the use of graphing. Nutrition goals, trends and concepts become more meaningful when children can see them plotted on a graph. Graph paper, colored pencils or markers and a ruler are all that is needed to complete the following bar or line graphs.

ACTIVITIES

▲ Using a completed one-day food record, explain how to count servings and graph daily food intake. After counting the number of servings from each of the five food groups and "extras," students can compare foods eaten to the recommended servings in *MyPyramid*. Ask them to explain what the graph shows about their diets. Based on the results, suggest they set personal nutrition goals.

▲ Have students graph personal nutrition or fitness goals. Examples include eating three servings of vegetables each day, limiting candy to one serving a day or bike riding at least twenty minutes daily. The vertical axis should include numbers from 0 to 10 (for number of servings) or 0 to 60 minutes (for minutes spent bicycling). Place a red dot or line at the level of the goal (if a bar graph, draw a red bar that represents

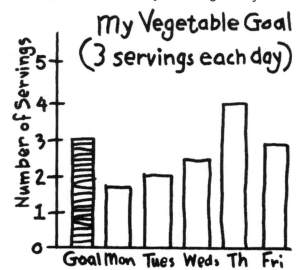

My Vegetable Goal
(3 servings each day)

Number of Servings

Goal Mon Tues Weds Th Fri

the goal). Underneath it, label it "Goal." Along the horizontal axis, write the days of the week.

Each day, keep track of how many servings or minutes. Plot results on the graph above the appropriate date. For line graphs, connect the dots to make a line. Ask students to explain their graphs and report progress in meeting their goals.

▲ Pick one food group and survey the class to find out how many servings from that food group they ate yesterday. Assign groups of students to graph the data in various ways. For example, ask how many servings of fruit were consumed. On the board, write down the number of servings eaten by each student. Ask one group to compare the number of servings eaten by girls compared to boys. Another group can compare fruit intake of students who ate the school meal versus those who brought a lunch from home. Still another can compare fruit servings by table or group. Other ideas include comparing students by birthday month, eye or hair color or whether their last name begins with a letter in the first or last half of the alphabet. (This activity is also a great way to reinforce skills in averaging numbers.)

Ask students to draw conclusions about the factors that might influence fruit intake in the class.

▲ EXTENSION IDEA: Involve the entire school in this activity, assessing food intake in other classes and grade levels. You may even want to challenge another class to a "good nutrition" duel, setting goals, graphing progress and rewarding completed goals with small prizes or incentives.

Create a Recipe

Devising a recipe gives kids a chance to develop measuring and writing skills, exercise their creativity and eat the results of their labor. They can also share their own recipes with family and friends or start their own personal "cookbook." Below are some simple ideas for recipe development where kids are sure to succeed.

Before you start, review the guidelines for safe classroom cooking advised in Appendix A.

For each recipe, provide a clean table with measuring cups and spoons, scale (optional), plastic knives and spoons, paper and pencils, plastic gloves, bowls filled with ingredients and individual plates or bowls for students to create their recipes.

Have students work in pairs, one as the cook and one as the recorder. After each recipe is complete, the children will switch roles.

YOU WILL NEED:

- Clean work space
- Measuring cups and spoons
- Scale (optional)
- Plastic knives and spoons
- Paper and pencils
- Plastic gloves
- Bowls filled with ingredients (see text)
- Individual plates or bowls

When creating a recipe, it is important to start small, measuring a small amount at a time and then adding more as needed. Remind students that they can always add more but they are not allowed to subtract. (It is not sanitary to dump ingredients back into the serving bowl.) Demonstrate how to accurately measure ingredients, using the plastic knife to level off the measuring cup or spoon. After students determine the "right" amount of an ingredient, the recorder's job is to write it down. Later at their desks, students can complete their recipes by adding instructions and illustrations.

▲ **TRAIL MIX:** Provide ingredients such as raisins, dried berries, other dried fruit (chopped, if needed), peanuts, almonds, pumpkin seeds, sunflower seeds, wheat germ and quick-cooking oatmeal.

▲ **YOGURT PARFAIT:** Use clear plastic cups to make the parfaits. Instruct children to layer their parfait as they wish, using such ingredients as fat-free lemon or vanilla yogurt, Grape-Nuts® or wheat germ, berries, banana slices and melon balls.

▲ **VEGETABLE SALAD:** Big on nutrition and easy to assemble, creating a vegetable salad recipe is one way to entice kids to eat vegetables. Include familiar and predictable ingredients (lettuce, tomatoes, cucumbers, carrots) along with more novel choices, such as sliced daikon radishes, jicama, sprouts, fresh spinach, colorful pepper slices, fresh sliced mushrooms, pea pods, green cauliflower and sliced summer squash.

▲ **PASTA SALAD:** This recipe is a great summertime dish. Offer some or all of the following ingredients: chilled pasta in at least two different shapes, chopped or grated vegetables (e.g., carrots, broccoli, cauliflower, sweet peppers, jicama, zucchini), grated parmesan or Romano cheese, sliced olives and mushrooms. Once students have assembled their salad, instruct them to mix it with reduced-fat or fat-free Italian dressing.

▲ **PERFECTLY PERSONAL PIZZA:** Students learn to create their own pizza recipe, perfect for a quick mini-meal or snack. Using English muffin or bagel halves as the base, spread with tomato sauce, sprinkle on spices, add toppings and sprinkle with grated part-skim mozzarella cheese. Examples of toppings include chopped onions, pepper rings, sliced black or green olives, mushroom pieces, broccoli or cauliflower florets, tomato slices, chopped turkey or ham and lean hamburger or ground turkey that has been browned and drained. Try spices such as oregano, garlic, basil, thyme, parsley or marjoram.

To cook pizzas, bake at 400 degrees for 8–10 minutes or broil for 3–5 minutes.

Calculating Daily Nutrient Intake
(ADVANCED ACTIVITY)

For students interested in calculating their precise intake of calories, protein, fat, calcium, iron or other nutrients, there are a variety of resources available.

▲ Nutritional Analysis Tool (NAT) is a free online diet analysis program that is based on the United States Department of Agriculture (USDA) food database and information from food companies. Developed for the Web by the Department of Food Science and Human Nutrition at the University of Illinois (Urbana–Champaign), the tool can be accessed at *www.nat.uiuc.edu/mainnat.html.*

▲ Students can assess their diets and physical activity using *MyPyramid Tracker*, an online tool based on the Dietary Guidelines for Americans 2005 and *MyPyramid*. The program can be accessed at *www.mypyramidtracker.gov*

▲ There are several programs available for purchase that analyze dietary intake. Most programs also compare intake to a standard recommendation based on age, sex and activity level. Data is usually presented in a variety of ways, including graphically. Although most programs are geared for students at the secondary level, many fourth and fifth graders possess the skills needed to use these programs. (See Appendix B, audiovisual resources, for catalogs that carry nutrient analysis software.)

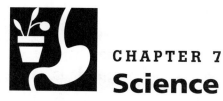

CHAPTER 7
Science

"Thank you for coming. I didn't know that (for) every pound we gain your heart has to beat an extra mile." —Mark

When my daughter was a first grader, she approached me about project ideas for her school science fair. I naturally thought of all the possibilities that related to food and nutrition science. The idea that sparked her interest the most was to survey her classmates and analyze their eating habits. By the time we finished this project, she had gained skills in a variety of subject areas. She developed a simple questionnaire that her classmates used to record their diets for one day, analyzed and compared their daily diets with the *Food Guide Pyramid* and presented her data graphically, using her best art skills to design, color and display her work.

Because nutrition *is* a science, the prospects for science activities are limitless. This chapter presents learning ideas in three areas: food in the body, the study of plants as food and how kids can use the scientific method to conduct nutrition research.

Food in the Body

Nutrition is the science of how the body uses food. Even young children can gain an appreciation of how food is broken down and used inside the body. The food we eat goes through five stages of processing: digestion, absorption, circulation, metabolism and excretion. Simple explanations with engaging experiments and activities will bring these concepts to life.

TASTE AND SMELL

Our experiences with food starts with our noses and tongues. The sensation of taste is actually a combination of smelling the food and using the taste buds on our tongues. While it was once believed that we use different areas of our tongues to taste different sensations — salty, sweet, bitter or sour — scientists now believe that we actually can detect most types of taste with most of our taste buds. In other words, the concept of the "tongue map" is outdated.

Scientists have also discovered an additional taste sensation named umami (pronounced oo-mommy) which is thought to be the savory or meatlike taste found in the chemical glutamate. Examples of the umami taste include meats, the seasoning MSG and aged cheeses.

ACTIVITY

▲ At snack or mealtime, instruct children to take a bite of one food and describe how it tastes. Next, have them hold their noses and take a bite of the same food. Ask them to describe the taste of the food and how it changed. Discuss how the sense of smell plays a part in detecting the flavor of foods. That is why the sense of taste is diminished when we are suffering from colds.

DIGESTION

Digestion is the process of breaking food down into millions of tiny pieces. Beginning in the mouth and ending in the toilet, food covers a route about 25 feet long, all inside the body! After the **mouth**, food travels to the **stomach** by way of a tube known as the **esophagus**. Most of the "action" of digestion occurs in the **small intestine**, a coiled-up organ that completes digestion and transfers nutrients through its walls to the blood stream. This so-called "small" intestine would stretch more than 20 feet if it were uncoiled! In the **large intestine** (larger around, but much shorter in length than the small intestine), water is added to waste products, making a paste that can be excreted.

While food is broken down somewhat by chewing and grinding, most digestion takes place by body chemicals. Chemicals known as **enzymes** break down food in the mouth, stomach and small intestine. Other

DIGESTIVE DIAGRAM

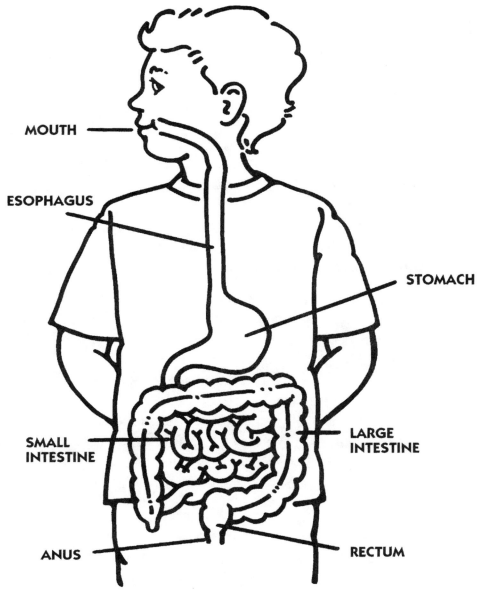

MOUTH

ESOPHAGUS

STOMACH

SMALL INTESTINE

LARGE INTESTINE

ANUS

RECTUM

chemicals include **acid** in the stomach and **bile** (which helps break down fat) released into the intestine by the gall bladder.

ACTIVITIES

▲ Trace children's bodies onto large sheets of paper, similar to the activity on page 66. This time though, students will be concentrating on how they look on the inside. Enlarge, reproduce or make page 103 into an overhead transparency. Ask students to draw and label the parts of the digestive tract on their life-sized silhouettes.

A digestive tract more than 20 feet long in a child four feet tall? How could that be? Using a tape measure and string, have students measure 25 feet of string. Using their life-sized body silhouette, ask them to "fit" the digestive tract into the one they just drew, affixing it with glue if they wish.

YOU WILL NEED:

- **Overhead transparency of page 103**

- **Large sheets of paper**

- **Tape measure**

- **String (25 feet per child)**

▲ Even as we are enjoying the taste of food in our mouths, digestion is beginning. As the teeth grind and crush the food, an enzyme in the saliva begins breaking down carbohydrates into sugar. To demonstrate this concept, pass out small pieces of saltine crackers. Read the label, pointing out that saltines are made from flour and have little or no sugar. Ask students to hold the cracker on their tongues without chewing or swallowing. What do they taste? After a few minutes, ask students whether the taste of the cracker has changed. Elicit possible explanations for this happening. Explain that the sweet taste means a chemical called an **enzyme** in their saliva has digested the starch to sugar.

Who was the first scientist to understand that body chemicals, not just mechanical action, are responsible for digestion? In 1822 an ambitious army doctor named Dr. William Beaumont was able to conduct digestion experiments on a living man! When fur trader Alexis St. Martin was shot in the stomach, he survived despite slim odds. But a small hole into his stomach never successfully healed, allowing Dr. Beaumont to conduct a multitude of digestive

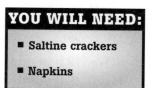

experiments and withdraw stomach acid for study. This fascinating story is told in *Dr. Beaumont and the Man with the Hole in His Stomach*, by Sam and Beryl Epstein (Coward, McCann & Geoghegan, 1978). Read this book to the class or encourage intermediate students (third through fifth grade) to read and report on it.

▲ The most slowly digested nutrient is fat. That is why a greasy meal can leave a person feeling stuffed for hours! One reason is that fat travels through the digestive system in big droplets or globules. When fat encounters the dark liquid **bile** in the small intestine, it is broken down into small droplets. Bile acts as an **emulsifier**, a substance that can break fats into small globules that will mix with water.

Using water, liquid vegetable oil and a raw egg yolk, students can observe how bile breaks down fat during digestion. An egg yolk contains the emulsifier lecithin. (Lecithin is often added to salad dressings and other processed foods because it breaks up the fat particles, resulting in a smooth product.) In a clear glass, mix 1 cup of water and 2 tablespoons of oil. What happens? Try stirring the mixture vigorously. Does the fat break down? Next, add the egg yolk to the mixture and stir. What happens to the fat

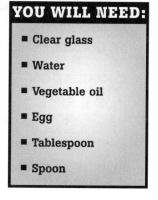

droplets? This reaction is similar to how bile breaks down fat in the small intestine. (Incidentally, egg yolks do not work as emulsifiers in the body since they are changed by both cooking and stomach acid before they reach the small intestine.)

ABSORPTION

After food is digested into small particles, it must somehow move from the digestive tract to the rest of the body. That movement into the bloodstream is called **absorption** and happens mainly in the small intestine.

The small intestine is made up of millions of fingerlike projections called **villi**. The villi are covered with a hairlike brush that traps the nutrients. The nutrients are then passed through the villi into tiny blood vessels called **capillaries** which eventually empty into the body's major blood vessels.

ACTIVITIES

▲ To explain the concept of absorption visually, use a sample of carpet to illustrate the surface of the small intestine. Each yarn fiber sticking out of the carpet is like a villus, ready to absorb nutrients and pass them into the bloodstream.

YOU WILL NEED:
- Carpet sample

Books for young readers that explore digestion include *What Happens to a Hamburger*, by Paul Showers (HarperCollins Juvenile Books, 2001) and *Burp! The Most Interesting Book You'll Ever Read About Eating*, by Diane Swanson (Kids Can Press, 2001).

CIRCULATION

How do nutrients find their way up to our noses and down to our toes? Every cell of the body requires a continuous supply of energy from nutrients and oxygen from the air we breathe. Oxygen and nutrients are transported to cells by **arteries**, while **veins** carry carbon dioxide and waste products out of the cells. This network of blood vessels, including the small, weblike, connecting vessels known as **capillaries**, make up the **circulatory system**. The circulatory system relies on a very important pump, the **heart**, to continually move blood through the body.

ACTIVITIES

The hard-working heart needs good care to work at its best. Eating a balanced, low-fat diet; exercising and controlling stress are all important heart-healthy habits to develop at a young age. Chapter 11 includes information and activities about the role diet and exercise play in keeping the heart healthy. *The American Heart Association* has a wide array of curricula designed to teach children about the heart and how to keep it healthy (see Appendix B).

METABOLISM

Once nutrients finally make their way to the billions of tiny cells that make up the body, they are used to supply the building blocks for energy, healing, maintenance and growth. Each cell of the body is like a tiny factory, taking the raw materials of nutrition and producing energy or growth and replacement parts. At any given moment, the cells of an active child are busy supplying energy to run at recess, creating new cells to make bones and muscles bigger, sending sugar to the working brain, and producing skin cells to heal a scraped knee.

Fortunately, the body does all these things without conscious effort. The only thing a healthy child really needs to think about is eating a diet that supplies the necessary raw materials.

ACTIVITIES

▲ What is hunger? It is the body's message to the brain that more nutrients are needed for growth, maintenance, repair and energy. By the time hunger sets in, the body's energy stores are running low and the ability to focus on tasks becomes difficult. To illustrate this point, ask children to respond to their hunger in other ways than eating: by reading, doing math problems, taking a walk, etc. (If possible, delay their lunch period by 30 minutes in order to carry out this experiment.)

Ask the children how they felt doing other activities when they were hungry. Were they able to concentrate? How were their energy levels? Their moods? Discuss the role that nutrition plays in learning. Point out that kids who skip meals, especially breakfast, often don't learn as well as kids who eat regular meals.

Ask students if they know what the word "breakfast" means (break the fast). Explain that a fast is a period of time without food. Elicit how many hours their bodies normally "fasts" from suppertime to breakfast.

On the board, write the sentence "Breakfast is the most important meal of the day." Ask students to write or tell whether this statement is true and why or why not. Encourage them to write about their own experiences with breakfast, including where and what they usually eat.

EXCRETION

The final stop for food is the excretion of waste products. Even the most nutritious food has parts that cannot be digested and used, such as fiber. After food leaves the **small intestine**, it enters the **large intestine** where water is added to form a paste that can be easily excreted. Other nutrient waste products are filtered through the **kidneys** and excreted through the urine (breakdown products of protein metabolism and salt, among others).

Plants as Food

Studying and growing edible plants is a wonderful way to reinforce nutrition and introduce children to scientific concepts and processes. Observation, prediction and data collection are skills gained by applying science to gardening. A "growing" classroom or home can be as simple as a few seeds planted in a milk carton or as elaborate as a greenhouse or large outdoor garden plot.

Young botanists should be encouraged to keep a journal when studying and growing edible plants.

PHOTOSYNTHESIS

A miracle really, life as we know it starts in the leaves of a plant. Using energy from the sun, carbon dioxide and water, **chlorophyll**-containing cells in green plants manufacture carbohydrate. Plants comprise the first link of the **food chain**, providing food energy for other living organisms, including people!

ACTIVITY

▲ To observe the effects of photosynthesis, start with a green potted plant. Instruct children to observe, draw and record how the plant looks. Place it in a dark closet. Continue to water regularly but do not expose to light. Every two days, bring the plant out briefly to allow children to observe and record the changes. How does the plant change? Ask children to draw a conclusion about the effect light has on plants. Explain that photosynthesis cannot occur, thus the plant can make no food, when light is removed.

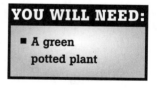

YOU WILL NEED:

■ A green potted plant

GERMINATION

Even when dormant for a period of years, seeds will sprout when given the right conditions of warmth and moisture. This process is called **germination**.

ACTIVITIES

▲ To watch germination in action, place dry beans in a clear glass jar containing a moistened sponge. The sponge will keep the seeds moist and hold them against the side of the jar where they are visible. Ask children to carefully record or draw the germination process in their plant journals, including any predictions they make about the process or how long it will take. (And later, notes on whether their predictions came true and why or why not.)

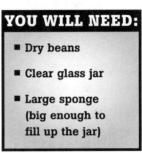

YOU WILL NEED:

- Dry beans
- Clear glass jar
- Large sponge (big enough to fill up the jar)

Ask if anyone's seed sprouted "upside down" or "sideways" (the answer should be NO). Elicit from the students how seeds know to sprout "right side up." (ANSWER: Seeds respond to gravity by sprouting root down, stem and leaves up. This concept is known as **phototropism**.)

▲ To grow edible sprouts, you will need small jars or clear plastic cups (baby food jars work great), clean 3-inch squares of nylon stocking, rubber bands and 1 teaspoon of rinsed lentils or dry beans. Place the seeds in the jar and fill it with water. Fasten the nylon square over the top with the rubber band. Let them soak overnight.

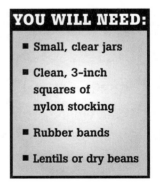

YOU WILL NEED:

- Small, clear jars
- Clean, 3-inch squares of nylon stocking
- Rubber bands
- Lentils or dry beans

The next day, drain off the water by turning the jar upside down until all the water shakes off. Rinse the seeds with cool water and drain again. Place the jar on its side in a dark place. Rinse the seeds twice a day and drain off water. Sprouts should be ready to eat in three to five days. For green sprouts, place them in a sunny window for one day. Eat and enjoy on salads, in sandwiches or stir-fried with other vegetables.

GROWING VEGETABLES

Potting soil or planting mix, empty milk cartons, and a sunny window (or grow light) will suffice for young gardeners just starting out. For classes who wish to garden on a grand scale, there are comprehensive programs available that assist schools in setting up a multigrade, integrated gardening curriculum. Before you embark on a school garden, be sure to check out the following online resources.

School Gardening Resources

▲ *schoolmeals.nal.usda.gov/Resource/farmtoschool.htm* (a source for school gardening resources from many states)

▲ *kidsgardening.com* (grant information and much more from the National Gardening Association)

▲ *www.edibleschoolyard.org*

▲ *www.lifelab.org/*

The activities below are designed to spark interest and encourage children to plant gardens at home. Most can be carried out with minimal time and expense.

ACTIVITIES

▲ Radishes are a great vegetable for the beginning gardener. Many varieties germinate in 4–7 days and are ready to eat in 25–28 days. First, fill cleaned half-pint milk cartons with potting soil. Read the seed packet instructions to find out the planting depth (usually 1/4 inch). Ask students to think of ways they can accurately measure the soil to arrive at the correct planting depth (a ruler or marked stick will work). Next, have students place four to five seeds in the soil (apart from each other), cover lightly and gently water. (To maximize drainage, poke a small hole in the bottom of the carton and place on a lid or in a tray.)

Encourage students to describe the planting process in their journals. Ask children to predict when their seeds will germinate and how the seedlings will look when they first sprout. Every day students can check on their plants and record any observations or changes. Keep plants moist but avoid overwatering.

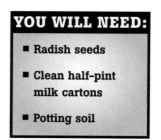
Once the seedlings sprout, encourage students to make daily or weekly measurements and/or predictions about the growth and record them in their plant journals. Results can be presented in a variety of ways — through drawings, tables or graphs, for instance.

▲ The radishes should be thinned to two plants per carton. They are ready to pick and eat when the roots become round and begin to pop up out of the soil. After harvesting, weigh the radishes and record that in the plant journals. Wash, slice and taste the radishes or use them to make one of the radish garnishes described in Chapter 10.

▲ A great springtime gardening activity is to "start a salad." Students can then take their seedlings home and plant them in small garden patches or in large pots placed on their decks or patios.

Materials to start a salad include an empty paperboard egg carton, potting soil and a variety of "salad" seeds. If possible, take the class on a field trip to a garden center or nursery to choose seeds for this project. Examples of salad greens include spinach, arugula, watercress and lettuce varieties such as romaine, oakleaf, butternut and redleaf. Fill egg carton compartments with potting soil and plant seeds according to package directions. When they have reached a height of 2 inches, send them home with a note to parents, encouraging them to transplant the plants outside or into a larger container. For easy transplanting, cut apart the

YOU WILL NEED:

■ Paperboard egg cartons

■ Potting soil

■ A variety of "salad" seeds (see text)

compartments of the carton, poke a hole in the bottom of each compartment, and place it in the soil, carton and all.

Encourage children to monitor the progress of their "salad" and record it in their plant journals.

▲ Just like all living things, plants have a lifecycle. Growing lettuce can make a fascinating study of the lifecycle of a plant.

As a class project, plant and grow lettuce in a large container in the classroom. Observe and record the progress of the plants and taste the lettuce when it reaches maturity. Allow at least one of the plants to "go to seed," a process where the lettuce will produce long shoots with flowers. Eventually the flowers will form small seed pods. (This process, from start to finish, takes a few months.) Start all over again by harvesting and planting the seeds — a perpetual experiment!

Ask students why plants "go to seed" and why harvesting seems to prolong the process. Discuss the ways other fruits and vegetables produce seeds. Ask students to bring in examples from home (e.g., avocado pit, cantaloupe seeds) and experiment with planting.

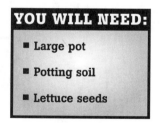

YOU WILL NEED:

- Large pot

- Potting soil

- Lettuce seeds

PARTS OF PLANTS WE EAT

The vegetables we commonly eat comprise a wide variety of "plant parts." There are six general classifications for edible plant parts including roots, stems, leaves, fruits, flowers and seeds. The activities below allow young botanists to classify, observe and eat various parts of plants.

ACTIVITIES

▲ Explain that vegetables can be classified by the part of the plant from which they come. The six general categories are roots, stems, leaves, fruits, flowers and seeds. (NOTE: The classification of vegetable as the "fruit" part of the plant can be tricky. Explain that a "fruit" refers to the edible part that grows from a flower and contains seeds on the inside. The "fruits" that lack significant sweetness are generally classified as vegetables). Brainstorm examples of vegetables in each category:

Roots: carrot, beet, radish (potatoes are technically tubers while onions are actually bulbs)

Stems: celery, asparagus

Leaves: lettuce, spinach, cabbage

Fruits: tomato, cucumber, eggplant, squash, pepper

Flowers: broccoli, cauliflower, artichoke

Seeds: corn, pea, green bean

▲ Take a field trip to a grocery market, farmers' market or produce farm. Encourage children to take note of the variety of produce they see. Upon return to the classroom, make a list of the observed vegetables and name the part of the plant each comprises.

▲ Bring a variety of vegetables into the classroom for observation and tasting. Include less common

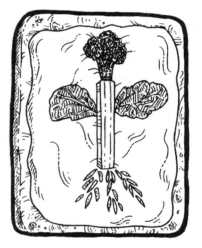

varieties, including daikon radishes, broccoli-cauliflower hybrid, Brussels sprouts, bok choy and kale. Provide hand-held microscopes that students can use to examine the vegetables.

Make "plant-part art" for a snack. You will need large, flat crackers; peanut butter or low-fat cream cheese; broccoli florets; celery sticks; lettuce leaves torn into small pieces and shredded carrots. Students will first lightly spread crackers with either cream cheese or peanut butter. Next, they will create a plant or garden design using shredded carrots for roots, celery sticks for stems, lettuce for leaves and broccoli for flowers. This is an amazingly novel (and effective) way to get students to eat vegetables!

Using Science to Answer Food & Nutrition Questions

Children can practice using the scientific method and also learn answers to food and nutrition questions at school or home. The scientific method involves formulating a **question**, developing a **hypothesis**, coming up with a **method** or experiment to test the hypothesis, evaluating the **results** and forming a **conclusion**. The hypothetical examples below illustrate how kids can apply this method to food and nutrition research. Students should also be encouraged to take the results of their experiments and use them to make recommendations for change.

Even very young scientists need to understand a few rules before setting up research experiments. It is important to get the permission of everyone involved, including cafeteria staff, administrators, students and parents. Individuals should not be pressured or forced into participating and individual results should always be kept confidential.

GARBAGE AS SCIENTIFIC EVIDENCE

Kids can monitor the cafeteria garbage to answer questions about what kids eat or throw away at lunchtime. The example below outlines one possibility for an experiment. Working in groups, students can come up with other ways of monitoring diets and influencing cafeteria choices by studying plate–waste.

Question: Which fruit do second grade students eat more of: fresh grapes or canned pears?

Hypothesis: Second grade students will eat more fresh grapes than they will canned pears.

Experiment: Empty lunch trays will be checked on two different days, including one day when fresh grapes are on the menu and one day when canned pears are on the menu. Students will stand by the area where second graders return their dirty trays and record whether the fruit was eaten, partly eaten or not eaten. The first twenty second graders who return their dirty trays will be studied each day.

Results: On the day fresh grapes were served, 12 of the 20 second graders ate the entire serving, 5 ate part of their grapes and 3 students did not eat any grapes. On the day canned pears were served, 6 of the 20 second graders ate the entire serving, 4 ate part of their pears and 10 did not eat any pears.

Conclusion/Recommendation: Hypothesis confirmed. Second graders prefer fresh grapes to canned pears. They ate more and wasted less on the day that fresh grapes were offered. The school lunch menu should offer fresh grapes more often and canned pears less often. Better yet, kids should get a choice of two or more fruits every day in order to eliminate waste and improve nutrition.

NOTE: Depending on the level of the students, the results can be manipulated mathematically, using graphs to plot raw results, or converting to percentages and presenting the data in a table or graph.

FINDING OUT ABOUT OTHER PEOPLE'S DIETS

Is it nosy to ask people what they eat? Maybe, but the government does it all the time when they conduct surveys of Americans' eating habits. Conducting nutrition surveys is a fun and informative way to learn about and compare the diets of different groups of people. Surveys can be descriptive, telling about the diet of a certain group of people (e.g., 8-year-old soccer players). Or a survey can be comparative, contrasting the difference in eating habits between two groups of people (e.g., soccer players versus piano players). The example below is a comparative study.

Question: Who eats or drinks more low-fat dairy products: third grade girls or third grade boys?

Hypothesis: Third grade boys consume more low-fat dairy products than third grade girls do.

Experiment: Design a simple checklist that includes the following foods: 1 cup low-fat milk (fat-free or 1 percent), 1 cup low-fat/fat-free yogurt, 1/2 cup frozen yogurt, 1/2 cup ice milk, 1 ounce low-fat cheese and 1/2 cup cottage cheese. Ask third grade students to check off each serving of low-fat dairy products that they eat or drink for two days. Remind them to pay attention to the serving size, making one check mark for each amount listed. (For example, if they eat 3 ounces of cheese at one sitting, that's three check marks) Do not tell them you are comparing girls to boys — they may make a contest out of it, which will bias the results. Instead, explain that they should eat and drink just as they normally do. Collect the surveys after two days.

Results: Fifteen girls and ten boys completed the survey. For the two days, the fifteen girls consumed 60 servings of low-fat dairy foods. The boys consumed 50 servings of low-fat dairy foods in two days. Using averages, the girls ate an average of 4 servings each in the two-day period (60 servings divided by 15 girls). The boys ate an average of 5 servings each in the two-day period (50 divided by 10 boys).

Conclusion: Hypothesis confirmed. Third grade boys ate an average of 2.5 servings of low-fat dairy products each day while third grade girls ate an average of 2 servings of low-fat dairy products each day.

MORE IDEAS

Once their minds are set in motion, students will enjoy using science to answer other food and nutrition questions. Encourage children to work cooperatively when planning and conducting their research. Perhaps the best gratification is that their projects can help initiate change in nutrition practices or policies.

Below is a brief list of other possibilities for nutrition research.

🍴 A study reported in the *Journal of the American Dietetic Association* showed that students ate more at lunch when they had recess before lunch. Test this hypothesis in your school, comparing two similar classrooms that have different recess/lunch schedules.

🍴 Working with the school cafeteria manager, set up taste tests with students for new nutritious foods offered by food manufacturers.

▲ Do a comparison study between kids who bring their lunches from home and those who get lunch at school.

▲ Nutrients that are commonly in short supply in the diets of pre-adolescents include iron, calcium, vitamin E and folate. Analyze and identify foods in the cafeteria that are good sources of these nutrients and create a poster to display the information in the cafeteria. A useful online resource for nutrient analysis is the food composition database from the USDA. You can access it online at *www.nal.usda.gov/fnic/foodcomp/Data/SR16/sr16.html.*

▲ If candy sales are a common school fundraiser, offer to study whether selling nutritious snacks (pretzels, nuts, raisins, trail mix, animal crackers, etc.) can be just as profitable.

▲ Poll teachers in the school to see how many teach nutrition in their classrooms.

▲ Design a study to test whether breakfast cereals with toys in the packages contain more sugar than cereals without toys.

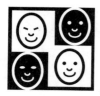

CHAPTER 8

Social Studies

"Your visit was FUN! Now I like vegetables more. My Mom and Grandma make Korean food — they make exotic animals! Since I was small my Grandma wanted to teach me it. Now they were impressed (by) what I learned!" — Tara

My childhood was filled with interesting food experiences, though I seldom appreciated their richness at the time. My grandmother of German descent prepared the most marvelous pastries, homemade noodles and *Kraut Bieroch*, a hamburger-cabbage mixture wrapped in delicious bread dough. My father, the son of a Greek immigrant, practiced his heritage by cooking wonderful Greek dishes. The week before Dad made *Kapama'*, a chicken-based tomato dish served with ziti pasta and cheese, the whole house smelled (some might say stink) from drying goat cheese, usually feta or kefalotyri.

A major goal of this chapter is for children to appreciate how dietary habits and traditions vary between individuals and cultures. Children will learn to identify and evaluate their own dietary customs and explore the food habits of people in other cultures.

A unit on corn stresses the role that this grain played in history and the continuing importance of corn in modern-day America.

Guidance is given for students interested in studying the problem of hunger in their community. Exploring the issues surrounding hunger allows students to learn, offer solutions and act to help those who lack access to nutritious food.

Identifying Individual Food Culture

Everyone eats, of course, but the what, where, when and even how of eating vary tremendously. Children don't need to go far to appreciate the diversity in food traditions. Even within a single classroom, children can discover great variety in family food habits and customs. Besides differences in ethnic origin and religion, families make choices based on personal preference and convenience. The activities below will help students identify their own traditions and perhaps start a few new ones.

ACTIVITIES

Identifying Food Customs: Ask students to think about the questions listed in Worksheet 8-1 concerning their food environments. Encourage them to design and share projects that explain their answers in a creative way (e.g., by writing and illustrating stories about their families' meals, designing skits, developing videos of their families' mealtime traditions or creating drawings, paintings or posters that depict their families at mealtime).

▲ **Carrying the Message Home:** Be sure that children share their work and ideas with their families. Invite family members to visit, share recipes, and describe their own childhood food experiences. Consider hosting a potluck and recipe exchange that features food favorites from each family (check local health regulations and policies first).

Blending Food Traditions: What happens when people from different cultures eat together? The book, *How My Parents Learned to Eat*, by Ina R. Friedman (Houghton Mifflin, 1987), explores how a Japanese woman and an American sailor overcome insecurities about their different eating customs.

How different cultures use the same staple food is explored in the "Everybody Cooks…" book series for young readers by Norah Dooley. Dooley's titles include *Everybody Cooks Rice* (Scott Foresman, 1992), *Everybody Bakes Bread* (Carolrhoda Books, 1996), *Everybody Serves Soup* (Carolrhoda Books, 2000) and *Everybody Brings Noodles* (Carolrhoda Books, 2002).

Another book that explores differing perceptions about food traditions is *Family Dinner*, by Jane Cutler (Sunburst, 1995). Geared for the intermediate reader, this is the story of how a modern-day family who doesn't "do dinner"

IDENTIFYING YOUR FOOD CUSTOMS

Everyone grows up with different food customs. The following questions will help you to identify your family's unique food culture.

1. Name and describe all the people in your family.

2. Does your family eat together? How often? Which meals?

3. Who decides what your family eats? Who shops? Who cooks? Who cleans up the mess?

4. Are there foods that your family especially likes to eat? Name and describe them.

5. What is your favorite food? Who makes this food? How often?

6. Are there special foods that your family eats on holidays or during religious celebrations?

7. Does your family sometimes eat foods that originated in another country? Name and describe them.

8. Describe a meal or celebration with food that was especially fun or meaningful (e.g., Thanksgiving dinner, bar mitzvah, birthday celebration).

9. Is there anything about your family's eating habits that you wish you could change? Describe the changes.

10. Fill in the blank: One tradition that I would like my family to begin is to _____. (Examples: eat breakfast together on Sundays, allow the kids to plan the menu once a week, turn the TV off at dinnertime, eat in a restaurant every other week, try foods from other countries once a month).

This may be duplicated for educational use.

reacts to the efforts of visiting Great-Uncle Benson who insists "you can't have a family without a family dinner."

Additional children's books with multicultural food themes are included in Table 8-1.

Table 8-1

CHILDREN'S BOOKS WITH MULTICULTURAL FOOD THEMES
The Ugly Vegetables, by Grace Lin (Charlesbridge Publishing, 1999) A tale about a little girl who thinks her mother's Chinese vegetable garden is ugly, especially compared to the neighbor's flower gardens. She changes her mind after her mother makes a delicious soup from the vegetables. Recipe included.
Good Morning, Let's Eat!, by Karin Luisa Badt (Children's Press, 1994) What do people in other countries eat in the morning? This children's book features descriptions and photographs of the breakfast habits of people around the world.
Is Anybody Up?, by Ellen Kandoian (Putnam Publishing Group, 1989) People in the same time zone (from Alaska to Antarctica) have very different ideas of what is good to eat for breakfast.
Potluck, by Anne Shelby (Orchard Books, 1991) This ABC book exemplifies a diversity of children and includes a wide variety of interesting foods such as asparagus soup, kale, peanut-butter pie, quiche, vegetarian stew, yams and yogurt and a zucchini casserole.
Bread is for Eating, by David and Phillis Gershator (Henry Holt & Co., Inc., 1995) All phases of bread production are presented with colorful characters and illustrations in a multicultural format. The phrase "El pan es para comer" (translation: Bread is for eating) is repeated throughout, with the complete song included at the end. This heart-warming story is presented in both Spanish and English.

Food Cultures around the World

Many different types and combinations of foods can be used to nourish the body. This becomes evident when studying various cultures and noting the differences in early native diets. But perhaps most interesting is the striking similarity in the nutritional composition of many native diets throughout the world.

Since the dawn of agriculture — roughly 10,000 years ago — people around the world have relied on a dietary staple rich in complex carbohydrate, most commonly a grain such as rice, corn, wheat, barley, sorghum, oats, buckwheat or millet. In some cultures, the primary staple is a starchy root such as potatoes, yams, cassava (tapioca) or taro. According to anthropologist Sidney W. Mintz, these carbohydrate sources provide more than half of the world's calories, even today.

In addition to this dietary core of complex carbohydrate, most cultures include a high-protein legume such as peas, beans, peanuts, chickpeas (garbanzo beans) or lentils. As Mintz explains, "This almost universal pattern in the diet of farmers is hard to explain; but whatever the reasons, it has been nutritively advantageous for our species."

Examples cited by Dr. Mintz include red beans and corn tortillas in Mexico; bean curd, mung beans and rice in Japan; wheaten bread accompanied by hummus (chickpea paste) in the Middle East; and, in Caribbean countries, rice or millet paired with red or black beans.

ACTIVITIES

▲ **Learning about Dietary Staples:** Explain to children the concept of "dietary staple," that is, the food that makes up the biggest piece of the diet, usually a carbohydrate such as grain or potatoes. Ask them why it is important to have a food rich in carbohydrates as the staple. Ask if they recall the body's first and most important need, nutritionally speaking. (ANSWER: Energy — see page 45 for a description.)

Discuss how cultures around the world have developed diets that are nutritionally similar, featuring grains or roots for carbohydrate and beans, lentils or nuts for protein. Elicit reasons why different cultures living far apart managed to develop similar diets. (Point out that early agrarians needed carbohydrates as a staple because their lifestyle as physical laborers required a great deal of energy.)

Ask students to think and list examples of ethnic diets that feature a combination of grains and plant protein. Common examples include tortillas and beans from Mexico, beans and corn (a mixture known as succotash) from American Indians, and rice and bean curd (tofu) in Asian cultures.

Explain how diets around the world now rely on a larger variety of foods and many cultures, like that of the United States, also rely on animal foods for protein, calcium and other nutrients.

It's hard to characterize the "American diet," since the diversity of groups that comprise our culture has resulted in an interesting dietary blend. (For instance, where else besides the United States can you find "taco pizza"?) Ask students how they think the rest of the world perceives the "American diet." (The probable answer is that American fast food, franchised through-out the world, is the perception of the U.S. diet by people in other countries.)

▲ **What's Your Staple Carbohydrate?** In this activity, students will keep a diet record for one to three days in order to identify if their diets have a staple grain or starchy root. Enlarge and reproduce the "What's Your Staple Carbohydrate?" Worksheet 8-2 on page 127 and pass it out to students. Students will count the number of servings from each grain or starch and record it on the worksheet. After they have completed the activity, ask them to draw conclusions and share with the class. While some may be able to identify one particular staple carbohydrate, many will notice that they eat a wide variety of grains and roots. Ask them how they think their diets differ from that of their early ancestors.

▲ **Identifying Grains:** Collect grain samples, including common varieties (rice, oats, corn, wheat), a few that are lesser known (barley, millet, quinoa,

WHAT'S YOUR STAPLE CARBOHYDRATE?

A staple refers to the food or foods that make up the biggest portion of a diet. Most early civilizations had a very limited diet that almost always centered on a staple that was high in carbohydrate.

Find out if you have a staple carbohydrate by keeping a record of what you eat for one to three days (using more than one day will give a more accurate picture of your diet). Record how many servings of carbohydrate-rich foods you eat in the proper spaces below.

NOTE: The standard serving size is listed beside each food. Be sure to take this size into account when counting your servings (e.g., If you eat 2 cups of pasta, that is equal to 4 servings).

WHEAT:
___ Pasta (1 serving = 1/2 cup) (e.g., macaroni, spaghetti, noodles)
___ Wheat Flakes Cereal (1 serving = 1 cup)
___ Bread (1 serving = 1 slice)
___ Bagel (1 serving = 1/2 bagel)
___ Hamburger Bun (1 serving = 1/2 bun)
___ English Muffin (1 serving = 1/2 muffin)
___ Flour Tortilla (1 serving = 1 10" tortilla)

OATS:
___ Oatmeal (1 serving = 1/2 cup cooked)   ___ Dry Oats Cereal (1 serving = 1 cup)

RICE:
___ Cooked Rice (1 serving = 1/2 cup)   ___ Crispy Rice Cereal (1 serving = 1 cup)

CORN:
___ Cooked Corn (1 serving = 1/2 cup)   ___ Corn Flakes (1 serving = 1 cup)
___ Corn Tortilla (1 serving = 1 10" tortilla)

POTATOES:
___ Baked Potato (1 serving = 1 medium)   ___ Mashed Potatoes (1 serving = 1/2 cup)
___ French Fries (1 serving = 12 medium)

OTHERS:
___ Barley (1 serving = 1/2 cup)   ___ Millet (1 serving = 1/2 cup)
___ Orzo (1 serving = 1/2 cup)   ___ Yams (1 serving = 1 medium or 1/2 cup)
___ _____   ___ _____
___ _____   ___ _____

After you complete this worksheet, answer the following questions:

1. Do you have one staple carbohydrate or do you rely on lots of different foods to supply your body with carbohydrates?

2. Why do you think people in early civilizations ate high-carbohydrate diets?

3. Why is it important for you to eat a diet high in the types of carbohydrates listed on this worksheet?

This may be duplicated for educational use.

triticale, etc.) and as many of the corresponding flour or meal products as possible. Set up a center where students can identify and label the grain and flour samples. Provide a mortar and pestle so students can experiment with grinding the grain kernels.

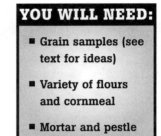

YOU WILL NEED:

- Grain samples (see text for ideas)
- Variety of flours and cornmeal
- Mortar and pestle

▲ **World Food Map:** Display a large classroom–sized map of the world, labeling it "World Food Map." Assign students to research one country to determine a common food or group of foods eaten in this country. (This can simply be an extension of an assigned report on a particular country.) They can find out this information by talking to people from this country; researching books, ethnic cookbooks, almanacs and encyclopedias in the library; calling or visiting restaurants that feature food from their assigned countries; or even writing to the countries' embassies or consulates. An excellent resource, complete with interesting and authentic recipes, is *The Multicultural Cookbook for Students*, by Carole Lisa Albyn and Lois Sinaiko Webb (Oryx Press, 1993). Another good source, written with the young reader in mind, is *The Kids' Multicultural Cookbook: Food & Fun Around the World*, by Deanna F. Cook (Williamson Publishing, 2003).

The following examples from the *Children's Britannica* illustrate one source of information that students can easily access:

> JAPAN: "Japanese–style meals include very little meat, butter and cheese. The chief food is rice served in a bowl and eaten with chopsticks. A great deal of fish is eaten, sometimes raw, and other foods include pickled vegetables, bamboo shoots, bean–curd soup, sweet potatoes and fruit".

> RUSSIA: "The chief item of Russian meals continues to be bread, which is usually of the "black" (actually very dark brown) kind. Other traditional dishes are *shchi*, which is a cabbage soup, and *kasha*, a grain porridge. Specialties of Russian cooking are *pirozhki*

(little meat pies), *blini* (pancakes), *borscht* (beetroot soup) and various forms of sour milk and cream."

ITALY: "The main meal, usually at midday, often begins with soup, which may contain rice, pasta or greens. This is followed by meat or fish, cheese and fruit. In parts of the Po valley, *polenta*, or cooked corn, is common and a lot of barley and chestnuts are eaten."

Give each child a 3" × 5" notecard on which to describe the assigned country's diet. They can do this in a variety of ways. They can write down the foods commonly eaten, draw a picture of the typical foods or an example of a meal, glue small pieces of dried food (rice, corn, beans, etc.) to the card or create their own representation of the country's diet.

Allow each child to give a short report on what he or she learned about the assigned country's diet. With the help of the students, find the countries on the World Food Map and tack the notecards on the designated countries.

LESSON EXTENSION: Ask students to find and share a recipe for a food commonly eaten in their assigned countries.

▲ Plan a class party or celebration that includes an ethnic theme and food. Examples include African dishes at a Kwanzaa celebration, Mexican food for Cinco de Mayo, or a potlatch to celebrate Native American culture.

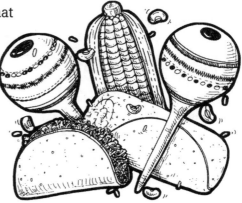

 Diversity in the School Cafeteria: Invite the school nutrition manager into the classroom to discuss how he or she plans menus that meet the needs and preferences of different ethnic groups in the school. For instance, some ethnic groups have a high incidence of lactose intolerance, which limits their ability to digest milk products. Other groups cannot eat pork or beef because of religious restrictions. Ask if there are ways that the school nutrition program accommodates these and other groups.

▲ Work with the school nutrition manager to plan menus and events that emphasize the ethnic diversity of the school community. Each month, a different grade or classroom could be assigned to develop a promotion for one ethnic group, complete with decorations, music, clothing or costumes, skits or dances and, of course, food.

▲ Offer to share recipes, food customs and traditions of various cultures with the nutrition manager. Suggest ways that the cafeteria can integrate these foods into the monthly menu, perhaps by offering a rotating "ethnic bar" on a regular basis.

> ## Check this out:
>
> *What You Never Knew About Fingers, Forks and Chopsticks,* by Patricia Lauber and John Manders (Aladdin Library, 2002)
>
> Starting with cavemen and moving throughout history, this delightful and humorous book covers the history of eating utensils and customs.

A Corn Unit

A grain with historical significance, the study of corn makes an ideal integrated unit. Besides discussing the nutritional contribution of corn, the history, modern-day uses and experience by different cultures make a fascinating study.

READINGS

Children will enjoy learning about the history and many uses of corn in *CORN: What it is, What it Does,* by Cynthia Kellogg (Greenwillow, 1989) and *Corn is Maize: The Gift of the Indians,* by Aliki (HarperTrophy, 1986).

High-quality color photographs show the modern-day production and harvesting in *Corn Belt Harvest,* by Raymond Bial (Houghton Mifflin, 1991).

HISTORY

Corn, also called maize, is indigenous to the Americas, comprising the staple food of many early Native American tribes. Corn spread to the rest of the world only after Columbus landed in the West Indies and obtained corn from the natives he named the "Indians." The earliest American settlers would have starved if the natives had not given them corn to cook, eat and grow. It was so valuable that the settlers used it instead of money to trade with the Indians for food and furs.

Most of the corn used by Native Americans was dried and ground into cornmeal using a flat stone called a metate, a job that was difficult and laborious. Today, powerful machinery in modern-day mills grind and process corn.

Eventually, the production and selling of corn became a way of life for many people who settled in what is now known as the "corn belt" of America (which includes Illinois, Indiana, Iowa, Kansas, Minnesota, Missouri, Nebraska, Ohio and South Dakota).

ACTIVITIES

Obtain several ears of field (also known as dent) corn from a local mill or farmer. Set up centers where children can explore various aspects of corn:

▲ First, children can remove the husks and silk from the ears, a process known as husking. Ask students if they can name the state known as the "cornhusker state" (ANSWER: Nebraska). Next, they can shell the kernels from the cob for use in the following activities. Ask children if anyone knows the name of

YOU WILL NEED:

- Several ears of field (or dent) corn
- Mortar and pestle
- Clean half-pint milk cartons
- Potting soil
- Fish emulsion

the machine that picks and shells large fields of corn (ANSWER: A combine).

Experiment with grinding the kernels. Provide a mortar and pestle, instructing students to grind one or two kernels at a time. (It's a difficult task!) Ask students to write or tell a story about how it must have felt to grind corn by hand, all day long for many days, like the Native Americans once did. (Some remote tribes still do!)

Native Americans and early settlers used all parts of the corn, including the husks and cobs. Husks were used to make dolls and art, braided into masks and stuffed into mattresses. Cobs were burned for fuel and made into corn-cob pipes. Ask students to brainstorm unique uses for cobs, husks and silk. Encourage children to use them in creative art projects.

Using empty half-pint milk cartons, potting soil and fish emulsion, plant three to four corn kernels in each carton. (Native Americans used fish to fertilize the soil when they planted corn.) Observe and record the sprouting and growth of the corn plants. (See Chapter 7 for more on growing plants.)

USES AND VARIETIES

It would be difficult to make it through one day without experiencing a food or product made from corn. In the average supermarket, there are thousands of food items that contain corn. Besides the obvious — cornmeal, corn flakes, corn chips, popcorn and grits — there are a multitude of products that contain corn syrup, corn oil and cornstarch.

The biggest use for the corn grown in America is animal feed. Corn is also used to make many nonfood items, ranging from tires and gasoline to glue, soap, medicines, cloth and many other products.

Although there are many varieties of corn, the three most common are field (also known as dent), sweet corn and popcorn. Field corn is used for animal feed, ground into meal and made into corn syrup, oil and starch. Sweet corn is a softer, sweeter type of corn that is eaten fresh on the cob, frozen and canned. Popcorn is eaten primarily as a snack food. Specialty corns gaining popularity include blue and white varieties, which are often made into gourmet corn chips.

ACTIVITIES

▲ Send students on a "corn hunt," either at home or a local supermarket, checking ingredient labels to find products that contain some form of corn. Divide the products into two lists, one that includes foods that are primarily made from corn (e.g., CornNuts, corn tortillas, Corn Chex® hominy) and those that have corn-based additives such as corn syrup, dextrose or corn starch (e.g., ketchup, pudding, soft drinks).

"CORNY" FOODS	
Main Ingredient	Corn Additives
Corn Flakes	Pudding
Corn Tortilla	Pancake Syrup
Hominy	Soda Pop
Popcorn	BBQ Sauce
Corn Oil	Gravy

🍴 Count how many items on the monthly school lunch menu contain some type of corn.

▲ Invite a corn farmer to speak to the class. Better yet, take a field trip to his or her farm. Other possibilities include visiting a mill that grinds corn or a factory that processes corn.

▲ As a class, have a cooking/tasting party of corn recipes that represent various cultures. Examples include corn tortillas (Mexico), corn bread (Native American) and ugali (cornmeal porridge native to Kenya). Good sources for authentic recipes include *The Multicultural Cookbook for Students*, by Albyn and Webb (Oryx, 1993), *Foods of the Southwest Indian Nations: Traditional & Contemporary Native American Recipes*, by Lois

Ellen Frank (Ten Speed Press, 2002) and *Spirit of the Earth: Cooking from Latin America*, by Beverly Cox, Martin Jacobs and Jack Weatherford (Stewart, Tabori, & Chang, 2001).

NUTRITION

While corn is rich in complex carbohydrates and a good source of plant protein, it is far from a complete or perfect food. In the early 1900s, people in the United States who relied primarily on corn as their dietary staple often developed the disease pellagra, caused by a deficiency of the B vitamin niacin. The disease had also been described in Italy and Spain as early as the 1700s. Interestingly enough, Indian and Mexican cultures who first soaked their corn in lye or lime avoided pellagra. (Scientists now understand that the lye reacts with corn to release the amino acid tryptophan, which the body can then transform into niacin.)

Using corn (or nearly any single food, for that matter) as an exclusive food inevitably leads to nutrient deficiencies. That is why *MyPyramid* is based on the premise that a variety of foods are needed for optimal nutrition.

Is corn a grain or a vegetable? That's difficult to answer, since Americans use it both ways, frequently serving frozen or canned sweet corn as a "vegetable." But from the standpoint of nutrition and botany, corn is best classified as a grain. (But why get picky?)

ACTIVITIES

▲ Students who enjoy library research can study and report on the disease pellagra, and how the U.S. Bureau of Public Health and doctors in the early 1900s finally solved the mystery of why people who ate mostly corn often developed this fatal disease. (A similar story to research and report is how a diet of polished rice led to the thiamin deficiency disease beriberi.)

▲ ENRICHMENT IDEA: Students can note the nutritional contribution that various grains make to the diet through careful label reading. Suggest that students check the labels of whole-wheat flour, corn flour and oat flour to compare the levels of fiber; protein; iron and the B vitamins thiamin, riboflavin and niacin in each product. Ask students to discuss which grain contributes the most nutrients to the diet.

YOU WILL NEED:

- Label information from whole-wheat flour, corn flour and oat flour

Helping Those in Need

Millions of Americans with limited resources go hungry each day. Faced with scarce pantries and empty refrigerators, many rely on community food banks and soup kitchens to make it through each month. Since food banks rely mostly on donations, the foods distributed through emergency food agencies are not always the most nutritious. According to one study, emergency food providers often fall short of dairy, fruit, vegetable and lean-meat items.

All ages are touched by this problem, including an estimated 2.7 million U.S. children. Hunger in America often goes unnoticed because few develop the telltale signs of severe malnutrition such as the wasted bodies and bloated bellies seen in drought- and war-torn developing countries. While few American children are on the brink of starvation, many are unable to perform or learn well due to marginal nutrition and transient hunger. Virtually every community throughout America is touched by the problems of poverty and hunger.

Children can become involved by learning, participating and offering solutions to the hunger problem in their community.

ACTIVITIES

▲ Invite a staff member from the local food bank, soup kitchen or other community agency to speak about the problem of hunger. Ask the guest to describe the extent and impact of hunger, dispel myths about people who are hungry, describe efforts underway to solve the problem and brainstorm with children ways they can contribute to the solution.

▲ Sponsor a schoolwide "nutrition drive" for the hungry, emphasizing donations of healthful nonperishable foods. Brainstorm lists of canned and dry foods that fit the guidelines of *MyPyramid*. Using the blank *MyPyramid* on page 52 as a model, create a drawing with examples of nutritious nonperishable donations. Send this list, along with information on the nutrition drive, home with all students in the school. Be sure to include information on how people who lack enough nourishing food can find help in the community.

Table 8-2

SUGGESTIONS FOR "NUTRITION DRIVE" DONATIONS	
FOOD GROUP	**EXAMPLES OF NUTRITIOUS NON-PERISHABLE FOODS**
Grains	Low sugar whole grain breakfast cereal, packaged dry pasta, whole grain crackers, brown rice, oatmeal, couscous
Vegetables	Canned corn, canned tomato or vegetable juice, canned green beans, canned carrots, spaghetti or pizza sauce
Fruits	Dried fruit, canned fruit (in its own juice), canned, boxed or bottled fruit juice, applesauce
Milk	Nonfat dried milk powder, canned pudding (made with skim milk), soy or rice milk in aseptic packaging, dried grated parmesan cheese
Meat & Beans	Canned meats such as chicken, tuna, salmon, sardines; canned or dried beans, peanut butter, packaged nuts, canned soups, stews and chili
Oils and "Extras"	Canola oil, olive oil, canned olives, fruit jam

▲ To promote the nutrition drive to the school and community, plan activities that increase awareness of hunger issues. Students can create and perform a skit on hunger, make posters and flyers, decorate food barrels or promote the drive through local supermarkets.

Enterprising young gardeners can raise money and awareness for hunger by selling vegetable and flower starts in the Spring. Start plants such as tomatoes, peppers, melons or flowers in small pots indoors approximately eight weeks before the sale. (See Chapter 7 for information on growing plants.) Tie the sale in with another event, perhaps a Mother's Day tea, music program, field day or other Spring school event. Working in groups, students can set up and decorate their plant stand, write an "advertisement" to send home to parents and take turns staffing the stand. Students will gain practice in running a business and develop math skills by changing and counting money.

YOU WILL NEED:

- Small pots
- Potting soil
- Variety of flower, fruit and vegetable seeds

If the school has a community garden, consider donating fresh vegetables to agencies that serve those who are hungry or homeless. Children may also want to plant and grow vegetables over the summer in their home gardens. Encourage donations of extra garden produce to agencies that serve the hungry.

CHAPTER 9
Performing Arts

"Thank you for the radish spinners,
They were just a treat.
Thank you for the pickle fans,
They were sour but good to eat.
Thank you for the orange peeled rose,
That looks pretty while standing in a pose."
     —Sweeta

Collaborating with a middle-school drama teacher proved to be a very gratifying experience. We worked with eighth grade drama students in the production of a nutrition play for elementary students. The idea was to motivate the younger children to try more healthful foods. I lent the nutrition expertise while teacher Adele White worked her magic, inspiring the students to create and perform a delightful 20-minute play. Using the costumed dog characters Sheggy Good-Grub (who eats well) and Sickly Spot (who subsists on candy, soft drinks and fried snacks), they enacted the consequences of nutrition choices in a play they titled "Sickly or Successful: You Decide."

The students performed the play for area elementary schools, leading the audience in exercises and stretching during intermission. The event was a huge success — the younger children were mesmerized during the play and nearly knocked Spot over (who transformed from "Sickly" to "Successful") after the play.

But the biggest surprise of all was the effect the process had on the actors. While eighth graders are not known for their great eating habits, these students actually began to take an interest in nutrition. (Granted, I did see cookies back stage a time or two.) The big surprise came when I arranged a pizza party (with healthful vegetable pizza) and they gobbled it up!

Through the process of acting, role playing and teaching others, students are able to internalize nutrition knowledge, making them more inclined to practice good eating habits.

Chapter 4 gives guidelines on setting up classroom dramatic play areas for children in the early grades. This chapter presents ideas on how to incorporate nutrition into performing art exercises and events. The children — so naturally dramatic and wonderfully creative — will inspire the best ideas. Please allow it!

Role Playing

Role playing in small familiar groups is a great way for children to "warm up" in a nonthreatening environment. Use realistic scenarios that allow children to think critically and solve problems. Stress that there are no right or wrong answers but instead, the goal is to practice making choices and explore the consequences of those choices. Use the ideas listed in Table 9-1 or create your own.

Creating Food and Nutrition Ads

Creating their own food advertisements helps children to understand the motive behind the messages that blitz their everyday lives. After reviewing the advertising techniques described below, set up activities that allow students to practice identifying these techniques in real ads. The final step is to use these methods to create positive ads touting healthful foods, nutrition, exercise or other health-promoting habits.

TECHNIQUES USED IN ADVERTISING

Advertisers use a variety of means to influence and persuade kids, many of which are cleverly disguised as games or promotions. The list below describes some of the ways advertisers commonly market products to children.

Table 9-1

WHAT WOULD YOU DO?

Working in small groups, encourage children to develop and act out solutions to the following scenarios.

- Your friend thinks she is too fat so she decides to go on a diet that she found in one of her mom's magazines. She wants you to go on the diet, too. How would you handle this situation?

- After school, you always feel so hungry. When your mom's not looking, you grab a bunch of cookies and go outside to play. Later, you don't feel hungry for supper. What would you do next time you're hungry after school?

- You like it when your Dad packs fruit, vegetable sticks and other healthful foods in your lunch. But the kids at school tease you about eating healthful foods, calling you "vegetable head." How would you solve this problem?

- Your friend says that a "Giggles" candy bar is healthful because the commercial on TV showed kids with lots of energy after they ate Giggles. He is now convinced that Giggles will give him energy, too. What would you tell him?

- On school mornings, you would rather sleep longer and skip breakfast. You really aren't that hungry when you first wake up, anyway. But lately, you have noticed that after morning recess, you have a headache, your stomach growls and it's hard to do your work. How would you solve this problem?

- You always have to rush to make it to afternoon soccer practice on time. You usually grab a can of pop and a package of potato chips to eat on the way. The problem is, your stomach often starts hurting in the middle of practice, especially if you have to run a lot. What do you think is causing your stomach aches? What changes could you make to solve this problem?

- Your best friend is a picky eater who rarely eats from the five food groups. You have noticed that he looks pale and tired and gets sick a lot. What could you do to help your friend?

- Your mom is a health-food nut. She is forever bringing home strange-looking vegetables with even stranger-sounding names, things like bok choy, kohlrabi and rutabaga! Worse yet, she expects you to eat them. You flatly refuse, saying you will not try anything that looks or sounds strange. Is there a better way to deal with this situation?

- Your big sister is pretty and popular but all she ever eats are salads and diet soft drinks. She says most other foods are "fattening." Is she right? What would you say to her?

- Your parents went out for the evening, leaving you with a teenage babysitter. She says you can have whatever you want for dinner, even candy! What foods would you choose?

▲ **Popular Characters or Celebrities:** Advertisers often appeal to the emotional attachment children have for a TV or movie character. Popular characters are licensed to sell a multitude of products — clothing, books, puzzles, toys and yes, even cereal and snack foods. Likewise, popular celebrities are paid millions of dollars in endorsements to peddle soft drinks to kids.

▲ **Constant Exposure:** Marketing has become very sophisticated, barraging children with nonstop messages. Beyond television commercials, children may also be exposed to in-school promotions and company-sponsored curricula, kids' clubs with special promotions and glossy magazines, and product placements in movies and sporting events.

▲ **Exaggerated Health Benefits:** The nutrition or health benefit of foods marketed to children are often greatly exaggerated in advertisements. Products that contain little fruit are praised by dancing fruit characters or shown with images of real fruit. Candy bars are played up for their ability to "energize." Highly sweetened cereals claim to be "part of a nutritious breakfast."

▲ **"Free" Toys:** Many food products appeal to children because they feature free toys or other mail-order giveaways. These products are often placed in grocery stores where kids will be sure to notice them.

▲ **Disguised Ads:** Advertisements in children's magazines are often cleverly disguised as comic strips, games or puzzles. Kids often think they are just another feature in the magazine.

▲ **Wearable Advertisements:** Many children are unknowingly walking ads for products. Shirts, jackets, backpacks, water bottles, sports jerseys and other everyday items often sport highly visible company logos.

Name _____

DISCOVERING THE MOTIVE BEHIND THE MESSAGE

This worksheet will help you to analyze how advertising and marketing influence the foods you buy (or ask your parents to buy). Use the checklist below to decide which methods are used to promote this product.

Food Advertised _____

Describe the advertisement (e.g., magazine ad, TV commercial, name or logo on a product, etc.) _____

_____

Check the categories below that apply to this food advertisement:

____ **Popular Characters or Celebrities** (Does the ad feature popular sports figures, celebrities or animated characters?)

____ **Constant Exposure** (Is the product marketed in many different ways? Do you often see this product promoted on television, billboards, magazines, clothing, etc.?)

____ **Exaggerated Health Benefits** (Do the ads for this product try to make you think that the food is nutritious or a good source of energy?)

____ **Disguised Ads** (Does this advertisement look like it could be part of the magazine? Is it presented in cartoon, puzzle or story form so it doesn't look like an ad?)

____ **Wearable Advertisements** (Is the company name or logo on something you can wear or carry such as a shirt, jacket, backpack or water bottle?)

Did this advertisement make you more likely to buy the product?_____

_____

Do you think the claims made by this ad are true? Why or why not? _____

_____

_____

This may be duplicated for educational use.

ACTIVITIES

▲ Ask children to bring in examples of advertising that use one of the techniques described above, including videotapes of commercials. Set up a center where students can identify and label the advertising technique, using Worksheet 9-1 as a guide.

YOU WILL NEED:

■ Examples of food advertising aimed at children

▲ For homework, ask students to watch at least one hour of children's programming on Saturday morning (excluding public television). Using Worksheet 9-2, have them keep track of how many commercials are for food. Based on what they know about nutrition, ask them to estimate whether the foods advertised are healthful (i.e., one of the five food groups, reasonable in fat and sugar content). Ask them to note if there were any PSAs (public service announcements) that promoted healthful eating.

▲ Contrast the goals of the advertiser with those of the consumer. Explain that companies are in business to make money and advertising is an important way to let people know about their products. Advertising also supports television programs and magazines. Discuss or debate the merits of advertising, posing questions like "What responsibilities do advertisers have?" or "Should advertising be banned?" or "Should companies who advertise concern themselves with children's health?"

▲ For information on how to write to food companies or television networks, see "Writing Activities for the Young Nutrition Advocate" on page 81.

CREATING A COMMERCIAL

Once children are familiar with the techniques used by advertisers, they can use this knowledge to create and perform their own 1- to 2-minute commercial for a nutritious diet, specific food or other healthful habit like exercise. Working in small groups, children can follow the steps below to create and perform their ad for the class, parents or other students. In

Name _____

TAKING A LOOK AT
SATURDAY MORNING FOOD ADS

To complete this activity, you will watch at least one hour of Saturday morning programming on a commercial network, such as ABC, CBS, NBC, Fox or Nickelodeon. Once you decide on the channel, do not switch networks until you have finished this assignment.

NETWORK WATCHED _____

DATE WATCHED _____

WHAT TIME DID YOU START WATCHING? _____

WHAT TIME DID YOU STOP WATCHING? _____

Every time you see a food commercial, make a tally mark beside the category below that best describes the food advertised.

_____ Candy

_____ Soft Drinks

_____ Sweetened Beverages (not 100% juice)

_____ Sweetened Cereal

_____ Corn Chips, Potato Chips or Other Fried Snacks

_____ Cakes, Cookies or Pastries

_____ Sweetened Fruit Snacks

_____ Other Sweetened Foods

FOOD GROUPS:

_____ Grains (e.g., low-sugar cereals, waffles, pasta, rice)

_____ Fruits (fresh, frozen or canned, 100% fruit juices)

_____ Vegetables (fresh, frozen or canned, vegetable juices)

_____ Meat & Beans (e.g., meat, fish, chicken, beans, eggs, peanut butter)

_____ Milk (e.g., milk, cheese, yogurt)

OTHERS:

_____ Combination Meals (e.g., children's frozen dinners)

_____ Fast Food Restaurants

_____ Public Service Announcements promoting good nutrition

_____ _____

_____ _____

How many total food advertisements did you see during the time you watched? _____

How many of these were for foods that you consider nutritious? _____

How many of these were for foods that are not the most nutritious? _____

Do you think there should be more advertisements for healthful foods on television?
_____

Why or why not? _____
_____

This may be duplicated for educational use.

some school systems, students may even have the opportunity to record their commercial as a Public Service Announcement (PSA) for local television or radio stations. The book, *Advertising: Media Story*, by Susan Wake (Garrett Educational Corporation, 1990), is a helpful tool for intermediate readers.

▲ **Brainstorm:** As a group, decide which healthful food or idea about good eating you want to "sell." Examples include a breakfast promotion, healthful snacking, a specific fruit or vegetable, "energy" foods, dairy foods for bone health, protein for a growing body or the importance of reading *Nutrition Facts* labels.

▲ **Create a Storyboard:** Working together, students will decide how to convince other kids to buy their products or take their advice. They will create a storyboard, which is the script for a commercial that contains both words and pictures. The storyboard tells all the specifics of the commercial, including details about music, actors, props, etc.

▲ **Assign Roles:** Once the storyboard is done, the group will decide who is responsible for each role. Students must agree on who will act, direct, be in charge of music, design props, etc.

▲ **Design Props or Costumes:** Students can create simple costumes or props on their own or enlist the help of parent volunteers.

▲ **Rehearse:** Students should practice the commercial until they feel it is polished enough to perform in front of others. They may also need to make minor adjustments to the storyboard or adjust the length of the commercial (it should not exceed two minutes).

▲ **Perform the Commercial:** Students can perform their ads for the class, other classes, the whole school during lunchtime or as part of a parent program. Videotaping the commercial gives students the chance to critique and enjoy their work.

▲ **Evaluate the Campaign:** Real advertisers want to know if their commercials work. Suggest students develop and pass out a simple questionnaire that asks the audience whether they are more inclined to try the food or suggestions just advertised.

Producing Skits and Plays

The possibilities are endless when it comes to developing skits and plays. Children can make and manipulate puppets, dress up as food or act as great chefs hosting cooking shows. The ideas in this section are meant to spark kids' creativity.

RESOURCES

Intermediate readers will enjoy the humorous account of the mishaps that occur during the class nutrition play in *Annie Pitts, Artichoke,* by Diane deGroat (SeaStar Books, 2001). Another excellent resource children will enjoy from the company *FOODPLAY* is the video *Janey Junkfood's Fresh Adventure.* An Emmy award winner, the program uses rap music, juggling, splashy graphics and dynamic young actors to communicate important nutrition messages. (See Appendix B for ordering information.)

SKITS

A skit is a short play with a simple message. Skits range from impromptu classroom exercises (such as the role-playing activity above) to productions that are elaborately planned and rehearsed.

At school, quick skits (15 minutes or less) can be used to promote an event or send an important message, as the examples below illustrate.

Work with the school cafeteria manager to promote a new food or menu. Perform a short skit in the cafeteria during each lunch period.

Develop and perform a skit about hunger and its consequences to promote a food (or "nutrition") drive for the needy (see page 136).

Demonstrate the link between nutrition and exercise in a skit that promotes a school fun run, walk, field day or other schoolwide athletic event.

To promote environmental awareness, plan a skit that emphasizes nutritious foods with minimal packaging. Demonstrate how certain food scraps can be recycled to make compost. (Students will enjoy acting as worms, demonstrating the breakdown of food to soil.)

PLAYS/VIDEO PRODUCTIONS

A play or video production is often longer than a skit, and usually involves more preparation, backdrops, costumes, props and music. Some ideas:

▲ *MyPyramid:* Create a play about *MyPyramid* such as "Chef Geometry Cooks *MyPyramid*," or "Food by Food: The Building of *MyPyramid*" or "*YourPyramid* or *MyPyramid*? Why one eating plan "does not fit all."

▲ **The Evening News:** Build a play or video production around the theme of a news broadcast. Feature a late-breaking segment about how "label reading before eating alerts kids to possible nutrition dangers," human-interest stories about kids who changed their lives through a more healthful diet, cooking segments, an opinion-based commentary on food advertising and on-the-scene coverage of the school cafeteria in operation.

▲ **Seasonal/Holiday Plays:** Put a nutrition twist on seasonal or holiday productions. Examples include "Goblins Who Gobble Good Goodies," "The Diet of the Pilgrims," "Frosty the Snowman Melts off Pounds," "How to Be Sweet without Sweets on Valentine's Day," "Why St. Patrick Likes His Greens," "Why Bunnies Don't Eat Chocolate" or "Nutrition and Your Teeth: Advice from the Tooth Fairy."

PUPPETRY

Children enjoy manipulating puppets and inventing stories. A classroom puppet area or theater is a good place for students to express feelings and create dialog. To encourage scenes about nutrition and fitness, include food props, puppet-sized jump ropes or personified food puppets. Kids enjoy making their own puppets, whether out of felt, paper bags, construction paper (finger puppets) or other materials. Resources on puppet making are included in Appendix B.

Children will enjoy creating a traveling puppet play on health and nutrition that they can perform for younger children.

Teachers or nutrition professionals can also learn to use puppets effectively. It doesn't take a great deal of skill to tell a story with a puppet or two. The amazing thing is that children will automatically be drawn to the puppet on your hand, even though they realize the words come from you. Speaking through puppets gives adults a chance to express ideas and knowledge in a new, refreshing way. Kids respond differently to a message from a puppet, too. (That's why puppets are often used to promote open communication with children who have been abused or have emotional disorders.)

Creativity Tips

Whether producing a commercial, play, video, skit or puppet show, the following ideas are fun ways to communicate good-food messages.

▲ Interject humor by using food as edible props. Use a banana for a phone, carrot or cucumber for a conductor's baton, or fruit as juggling balls. An even more comical approach is for the characters to eat the props as they use them!

▲ A nice addition to a production is the use of poems about food or silly nutrition songs set to common tunes.

▲ Puppets can be used as props within a play or video production. Food puppets can hover over a character's head, playing the role of the "conscience," which tries to convince kids why they should be eaten. A puppet show can also serve as an effective "play within a play," or as a television show or commercial set within a play.

▲ Kids can play the part of life-sized food models. To help children "feel" the part, have a tasting party using real foods. As children taste apples, asparagus, French bread or farmer's cheese, have them imagine how the texture, appearance and flavor would transfer into a character role. An orange, for instance, may decide to act in a very sour manner, the cheese wedge might portray a mellow character or the grapes may decide to act very sweet.

Create a "Madame Food-sauds" Wax Museum

One idea is to create a museum of food using real children as "waxed" fruits and vegetables. Assign each child a specific fruit or vegetable and instruct them to research interesting facts about their produce, including how they grow, major nutrients, the best way to prepare them and maybe even a short recipe. A great resource for this information is the Dole 5-A-Day Web site located at *www.dole5aday.com*.

Children can put together costumes that represents their fruits or vegetables. To create the effect of a wax museum, have them stand perfectly still with paper "on" switches on the floor near where they are standing. To activate the wax figure, visitors will step on the switch. The fruit or vegetable then begins the presentation on how it grows, why it is good to eat, etc. This is a great presentation to do for parents' night at school.

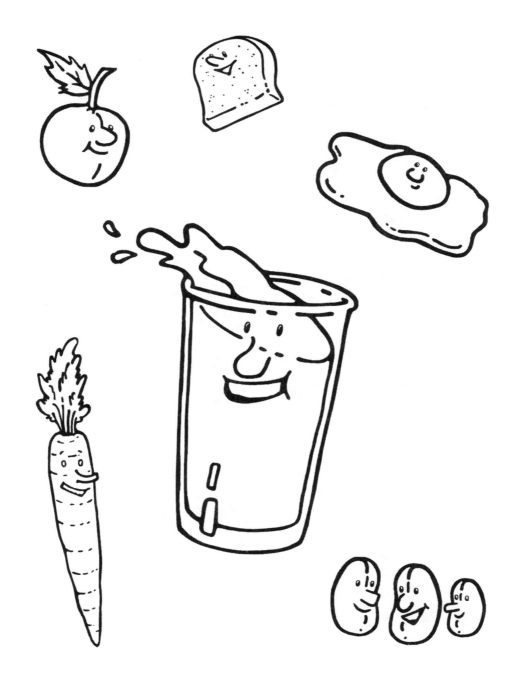

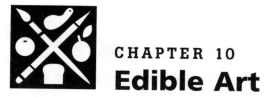

CHAPTER 10

Edible Art

"Thank you for showing us how to make those fruit 'sculptures.' Last night I asked my mom to buy some oranges and she did. I tried to make a rose but I didn't do it but I did better." —Krystal

More than mere cooks, many chefs are artists in their own right. Instead of paints and canvas or chisels and bronze, their medium is food and their tools are kitchen gadgets and knives. Like artists who make oceanside sand sculptures, the art created by chefs is transient, but beautiful nonetheless.

These edible art ideas will capture the imagination of children as they delight in playing with their food. Some of the activities are easy while others require more practice. They are all designed with safety in mind — they can be completed using plastic serrated knives and other tools that are safe when handled properly.

Aside from the artistic merits of their work, children will also enjoy eating their creations!

As with any food activity, be sure to review the safety and sanitation guidelines outlined in Appendix A before beginning.

Zigzag Fruits

YOU WILL NEED:

- 1 piece of fruit per child (oranges, lemons, grapefruits, firm kiwifruit or small melons)
- plastic ridged or semi-ridged knives
- clean work surface and hands

DIRECTIONS:

Cut a zigzag pattern (see diagram) completely around the circumference of the fruit, inserting knife to approximately the center of the fruit. For better control, instruct children to hold the knife approximately 1 to 1–1/2" from the tip as they cut.

Pull fruit apart to expose two fancy "crowns," suitable for a garnish or fancy snack.

Chef Tip: Different fruits can be stacked on top of each other to form a flower.

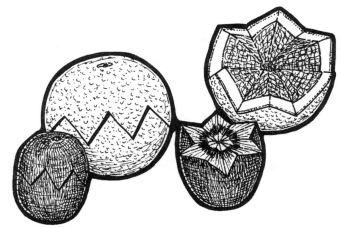

Creative Kebabs

Suggested Fruits: slices/chunks of banana, kiwi, apple, pear, pineapple, melon, orange wedges, star fruit, papaya, strawberries (a spritz of orange or lemon juice will keep fruits such as bananas, apples, and kiwi from turning brown)

Suggested Vegetables: Slices/chunks of radishes, cucumber, cherry tomatoes, carrots, broccoli or cauliflower florets, mushrooms, pea pods, summer squash

DIRECTIONS:

Create either fruit or vegetable kebabs by threading them onto a wooden skewer. Encourage creative use of color, design and patterning. Discuss how kebabs could be arranged artfully on a platter, placing a bowl of suggested dip in the center.

Chef Tip: Make a bouquet-type display of vegetables by inserting three or four kebabs into a raw potato half. For a fruit bouquet, insert three or four fruit kebabs into a melon half.

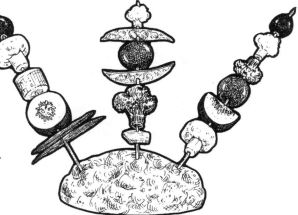

Food "Fans"

YOU WILL NEED:

- soft fruit or vegetable such as a fresh peach half, ripe fresh pear half, whole strawberry or a large pickle or cucumber half for each child

- plastic ridged or semi-ridged knives

- clean work surface and hands

DIRECTIONS:

Place food on work surface so that it is stable (cut "rounded" foods in half to prevent them from rolling). Starting approximately one-half inch from the top, make a cut completely through the fruit or vegetable (see diagram). Make several cuts, parallel to the first one. Press down and "fan out."

Chef Tip: Cucumbers have a great success rate for this garnish. Try making the cuts at an angle across the cucumber for a different effect.

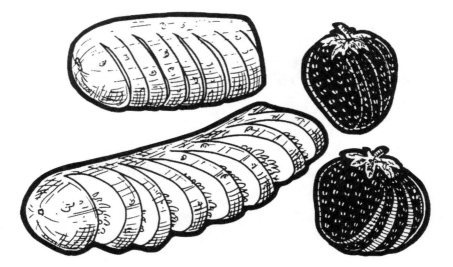

Baby Goose in a Nest

YOU WILL NEED:

- small or "baby" crooked neck squash, whole cloves, alfalfa sprouts, orange
- plastic ridged or semi-ridged knives
- clean work surface and hands

DIRECTIONS:

Cut the orange in half, using the zigzag cut described on page 154. Carefully scoop and/or cut the edible contents out of the orange half, making sure to leave the peel in one piece. Create a "nest" by filling the orange peel with alfalfa sprouts.

Next, cut the squash off about an inch below the "neck." Insert whole cloves near the stem to make eyes (see diagram). Nestle the goose head and neck into the sprouts, so it appears the goose is poking out from his nest. If you wish, place two or three squash geese in each nest.

NOTE: Don't be wasteful! Be sure to eat the orange that was scooped out of the peel. The bottom portion of the squash can be sliced and eaten raw, cooked or used in another project.

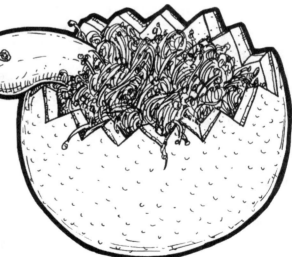

Chef Tip: Use small radishes or jelly beans for "eggs" in the nest.

Radish Garnishes

Radishes are frequently used in garnishing because they are inexpensive, colorful and versatile. They are also easy to grow — see Chapter 7, page 111 for instructions. Three examples of radish garnishes are described below.

YOU WILL NEED:

- whole radishes, thinly sliced radishes, cherry tomatoes, lettuce leaves, whole cloves, uncooked spaghetti
- plastic ridged or semi-ridged knives
- clean work surface and hands

DIRECTIONS:

Radish Jacks: To make a jack, use two thin slices of radish. Make a single slit to the center point of each slice. Slip cut ends together to make a jack. To make a display of jacks and a ball, make several radish jacks and use a plump, round radish for the "ball."

Radish Caterpillar: Using thinly sliced radishes, arrange slices on a lettuce leaf, as shown in diagram. For a head, use a cherry tomato half with cloves for eyes and small pieces of broken spaghetti for antennae. Use the same technique to make caterpillars out of sliced carrots or small cucumbers.

Chef Tip: White icicle radishes work great because they are long. Watch out though — these can taste very hot and spicy!

Radish Mouse: Use a large whole radish with the root (which becomes the tail) still attached. Trim the stem, leaving a small stub for the nose. Use two thin radish slices from another radish for the ears. Make small slits on top of the "head" and insert ears. Use whole cloves for eyes and small pieces of broken spaghetti for whiskers.

Sandwich Art

Use the following ideas to turn sandwiches into artwork that looks back at you!

HOAGIE FACES

YOU WILL NEED:

- hoagie buns, sliced low-fat cheese, lean luncheon or deli meat, shredded carrots, lettuce or sprouts, olives, cherry tomatoes
- miscellaneous condiments (mustard, reduced-fat mayonnaise, etc.)
- toothpicks (or broken spaghetti pieces)
- clean work surface and hands

DIRECTIONS:

Make hoagie sandwich, using desired ingredients. On one end of the sandwich, use toothpicks or broken spaghetti pieces to position olives for eyeballs, and cherry tomato for nose. Arrange shredded carrots, lettuce or sprouts on top for hair (see diagram). If desired, stick a small piece of lunch meat out of the "mouth" for a tongue. NOTE: Be sure to remove all toothpicks before eating!

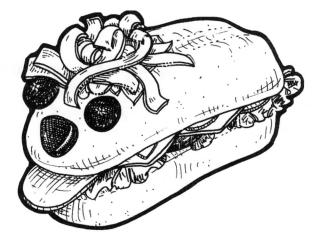

SMILING BURRITOS

YOU WILL NEED:

- corn or flour tortilla, refried beans, grated part-skim mozzarella cheese, black olives, cherry tomato, kidney or black beans, orange wedges

- salsa (optional)

- microwave-safe plate

- spoon

- clean work surface and hands

DIRECTIONS:

Spread refried beans on tortilla. Use remaining ingredients to make a smiling face: cheese for hair, olives for eyes, a cherry tomato nose and bean smile. Microwave on high for 1 minute. Place orange wedges beside the burrito for ears. If desired, serve with salsa.

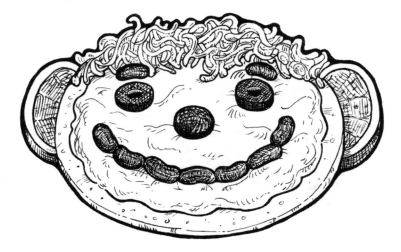

TUNA MANDARIN ROLL-UPS

Spice up ordinary tuna salad with curry powder and sweet, colorful Mandarin oranges.

YOU WILL NEED:

- 1 can (12 ounces) solid white albacore tuna in water, drained
- 1/4 cup reduced-fat mayonnaise
- 1/4 teaspoon curry powder
- 1 can (11 ounces) Mandarin orange segments, drained
- 1/3 cup finely chopped celery
- 4 medium flour tortillas
- 2 cups lettuce or baby spinach leaves
- Measuring cups and spoons, fork, spoon, mixing bowl, plates
- clean work surface and hands

DIRECTIONS:

In medium bowl, use fork to combine tuna, mayonnaise and curry powder. Mix well. Stir in oranges and celery. Spread 1/2 cup tuna mixture onto each tortilla to within 1 inch of edge; top with 1/2 cup lettuce. Roll up; serve immediately.

Makes 4 servings.

Courtesy of the
Canned Food Alliance
www.mealtime.org.

PIZZA FACES

- English muffins or bagel halves (split open), prepared pizza or spaghetti sauce, grated part-skim mozzarella cheese, vegetables such as sliced olives, sliced mushrooms, red pepper rings, chopped onions and broccoli florets
- spoons
- clean work surface and hands

DIRECTIONS:

Spread English muffin half with pizza sauce and top with mozzarella cheese. Using the vegetables, create a "face" design. Broil 3-4 minutes or until cheese is golden and bubbly.

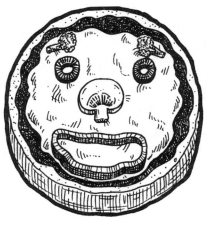

Chef Tip: Adapt this activity for special holidays. Make Jack-O'-Lantern, Santa, Cupid or Leprechaun pizza faces!

FRESH FACES

YOU WILL NEED:

- English muffins (split open) or toaster waffles, peanut butter or reduced fat cream cheese, pineapple tidbits, sunflower seeds, raisins, berries and banana slices
- plastic knives
- clean work surface and hands

DIRECTIONS:

Spread muffin half or toasted waffle with peanut butter or cream cheese. Using remaining ingredients, make a face or other art design.

Bread Dough Art

Using bread dough, children can create virtually any shape, letter, animal or design that they wish. It's as versatile as clay and a lot more delicious!

YOU WILL NEED:

- frozen bread dough (whole wheat is preferable), unbaked roll or bread dough from the school cafeteria or bread dough from scratch
- cookie sheet and parchment baking paper
- clean work surface and hands

DIRECTIONS:

If dough is frozen, thaw beforehand. On a floured surface, divide dough into individual portions. Pass out to children, instructing them to roll, knead and shape dough into desired shapes. Place on cookie sheet lined with parchment baking paper, labeling each child's creation. Preheat oven to 375°F. Let rise, uncovered, for 15–20 minutes in a warm, draft-free place. Bake bread on center shelf of oven for 15–20 minutes (until golden brown). Cooking time will vary depending on shape and thickness of art.

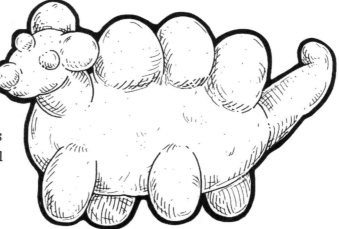

OPTIONAL: Discuss the scientific principles involved in bread baking, including how yeast causes bread to rise and predictions about how the art will change during the baking process.

Very Berry Frozen Pops

These colorful, tasty pops can be garnished with fresh berries or a fanned-out strawberry from page 156.

from page 156.

YOU WILL NEED:

- 1 cup flavored low-fat yogurt (try blueberry, vanilla, or lemon)
- 1 cup fresh or thawed frozen berries (blueberries, strawberries, raspberries, or a mixture of all three)
- 4 3-ounce paper cups
- 4 plastic spoons
- Measuring cup, mixing bowl, fork or masher
- clean work surface and hands

DIRECTIONS:

In medium bowl, mash berries with a fork or masher until they are a smooth consistency. Add the yogurt and mix well. Divide the mixture evenly between the four paper cups. Stick a plastic spoon in the middle. Freeze for two hours or until the pops are solid. Peel off the paper cup and enjoy!

Makes 4 frozen pops.

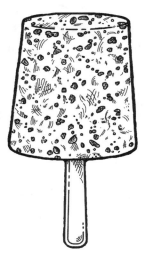

Yummy Pumpkin Softies

These delicious soft cookies are packed with nutrition. Kids can use dried fruit and nuts to create their own "designer" cookies.

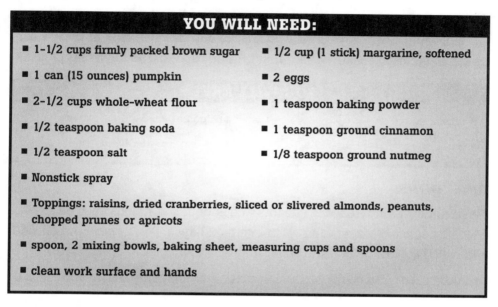

YOU WILL NEED:

- 1-1/2 cups firmly packed brown sugar
- 1 can (15 ounces) pumpkin
- 2-1/2 cups whole-wheat flour
- 1/2 teaspoon baking soda
- 1/2 teaspoon salt
- Nonstick spray
- Toppings: raisins, dried cranberries, sliced or slivered almonds, peanuts, chopped prunes or apricots
- spoon, 2 mixing bowls, baking sheet, measuring cups and spoons
- clean work surface and hands

- 1/2 cup (1 stick) margarine, softened
- 2 eggs
- 1 teaspoon baking powder
- 1 teaspoon ground cinnamon
- 1/8 teaspoon ground nutmeg

DIRECTIONS:

Preheat oven to 350°F. In mixing bowl, beat together sugar and margarine until creamy. Add pumpkin and eggs; beat well. In medium bowl, combine flour, baking powder, baking soda, cinnamon, salt and nutmeg; add to pumpkin mixture, mixing until dry ingredients are moistened. Lightly spray baking sheets with nonstick spray. Drop dough by rounded measuring tablespoonfuls onto prepared pans. Smooth tops of dough with back of spoon and decorate with dried fruits and nuts to make flowers, faces or other fun patterns. Bake 15 to 18 minutes or until bottoms are golden brown (lift gently with a spatula to check). Remove to wire racks; cool completely. **Makes about 3-1/2 dozen.** Courtesy of the Canned Food Alliance *www.mealtime.org.*

Cookie Cutter Fun

Cookie cutters can be used with food in many imaginative ways. Designs are especially fun when they complement thematic units or parties.

You don't even need actual cookie cutters — hunt the classroom or playroom for interesting plastic toys of varying shapes and sizes. As long as objects can be sanitized in hot, soapy water, they can be used for the following projects.

YOU WILL NEED:

- cookie cutters
- foods of choice (see directions)
- plastic ridged or semi-ridged knives
- clean work surface and hands

DIRECTIONS:

Fun-Shaped Sandwiches: Cut sandwiches with soft fillings such as cheese, peanut butter or tuna salad into fun shapes. Don't waste the outside edges — they can be cut into small finger sandwiches.

Breakfast Art: Use cookie cutters to make fun-shaped pancakes, waffles or French toast.

Cheese Shapes: Cut cheese slices into various shapes and arrange on a platter with crackers. Or, melt cheese shapes onto dark bread or toast to make unique open-faced toasted cheese sandwiches. (Children this age require supervision when using the broiler or microwave oven.)

Contrasting Cutouts: Using either light and dark breads (light rye and pumpernickel work well) or white and orange cheeses, create contrasting designs with cookie cutters. Carefully cut identical sections out of both slices of cheese or bread. Insert the dark cutout into the light piece and the light cutout into the dark piece (see diagram).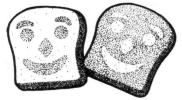

Indentations: On the top of bread, sandwiches, pancakes or sliced cake, press cookie cutter lightly until an indentation is visible.

Expanding on Edible Art

The following ideas can be assigned as homework or included as suggestions in a parent newsletter.

▲ At home, encourage children to garnish a serving platter, salad bowl or individual plates as a way to make family dinners extra special.

▲ Older children may want to host or "cater" an event for their friends. Birthday or holiday parties, post-game get-togethers or even "break the boredom" events are all chances for kids to impress their friends with their food savvy.

▲ Snacktime becomes learning and fun time when students prepare food in fancy ways. Children may actually eat a more varied diet when they have a hand in making it.

At school, students can make fancy garnishes for the cafeteria serving line or self-service variety bars.

▲ Invite a local chef to come to the classroom and teach students additional garnishes and cooking skills, expose children to careers in the culinary field and reinforce nutrition concepts.

▲ Encourage children to expand their culinary skills by checking out one of the kids' cookbooks or garnishing books listed in Appendix B.

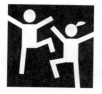

CHAPTER 11

Physical Education

If I were a car, I wouldn't get far
Without some gas, so please pass
Some human fuel (known as food),
To fill my tank and improve my mood!
                — *CLE*

Food is only one part of the fitness equation. The optimal growth and development of young bodies requires movement, play and exercise. A successful physical fitness program emphasizes fun, fitness and the attainment of life skills.

Children who are active feel better, have more energy and even learn more easily than their sedentary peers. A strong physical education program, along with a solid nutrition program, boosts the entire school learning environment. Children in good physical condition bring more focus, stamina and creativity to the classroom.

Fit Kids Are Smarter Kids

There is a distinct relationship between academic achievement and physical fitness, according to a study by the California Department of Education. In the study, reading and math scores were matched with fitness scores of 353,000 fifth graders, 322,000 seventh graders and 279,000 ninth graders. The key findings:

• Higher achievement was associated with higher levels of fitness at each of the three grade levels measured.

• The relationship between academic achievement and fitness was greater in math than in reading, particularly at higher fitness levels.

• Students who met minimum fitness levels in three or more physical fitness areas showed the greatest gains in academic achievement at all three grade levels.

Nutrition principles are naturally integrated into the study and practice of physical education. This chapter includes activities which reinforce the role diet and exercise play in heart health, the importance of goal setting when targeting health behaviors, the best foods to eat for sports and play, active games that reinforce nutrition knowledge and secrets from one teacher who integrates walking into all aspects of her curriculum.

Taking Care of the Hard-Working Heart

The strongest muscle in the body, the heart pumps an average of 2,000 gallons of blood each day. Because it is a muscle, the heart becomes stronger and more efficient when it is exercised regularly.

> **E**very day, kids should engage in at least one hour of physical activity such as P.E., organized sports or active play.

Diet also plays a vital role in keeping the heart healthy. While nutrition scientists continue to search for definitive answers about diet and heart health, they do know that a high intake of cholesterol, saturated fat and trans fat places many people at increased risk for heart disease. When the concentration of cholesterol in the blood runs consistently high, fatty deposits eventually build up in the **coronary arteries**, the blood vessels that supply the heart with oxygen and nutrients. When a coronary artery becomes completely blocked with fat, the blood supply to that section of the heart muscle is shut off, resulting in the life-threatening event known as a "heart attack."

Limiting fat is only one piece of a heart smart lifestyle, though. Eating an overall well-balanced diet — rich in high-fiber grains, beans, fruits and vegetables — lowers the risk of heart disease.

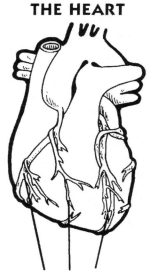

THE HEART

CORONARY ARTERIES

Also vital to heart health are lifetime habits that include regular exercise, relaxation, a tobacco-free lifestyle and the control of blood pressure.

While it is the rare child who will experience coronary heart disease in youth, autopsy studies demonstrate that the process leading to fatty arteries begins in childhood. Clearly, the best "cure" for heart disease involves adopting healthful habits early on.

Table 11-1

FAT FACTS

▲ Fat is essential to health, development and growth. In spite of all the negative press, some fat is needed, both on the body and in the diet:

▸ In the body, fat serves as a shock absorber that protects internal organs, aids in temperature regulation, provides insulation, serves as an energy reservoir and comprises an important part of the cell membrane.

▸ In the diet, fat provides the essential fatty acids linoleic and linolenic acids. Dietary fat also aids in the transport and absorption of the fat–soluble vitamins (A, D, E and K).

▸ Fat plays an important role in promoting growth and development in infants. Breast milk – nature's perfect food for babies – derives more than half of its calories from fat and is high in cholesterol as well.

▸ Fat tastes good and provides a feeling of satisfaction. Since fat is digested more slowly than carbohydrate or protein, it delays feelings of hunger between meals.

▲ Too much fat — both in the diet and on the body — creates problems for a large percentage of Americans. The rate and severity of obesity continues to rise for both children and adults (in spite of a multibillion dollar weight-loss industry).

▲ Fat is "fattening" in the sense that it contains nine calories per gram, while the other energy nutrients — carbohydrate and protein — each contain four calories per gram.

▲ Obesity is associated with many chronic health problems, including high blood pressure, mechanical stress on the joints, diabetes, heart disease and certain types of cancer.

(Table 11-1 continues on next page)

Table 11-1 (continued)

▲ A high level of cholesterol in the blood is a major risk factor for coronary artery disease. A blockage in an artery leading to the brain can cause a stroke, while a blockage in the coronary arteries leads to heart attack.

▲ It is ironic and confusing that dietary cholesterol has only a moderate effect on blood cholesterol levels. The real culprit in elevated blood cholesterol levels is the amount of saturated fat eaten. The types of fat are briefly described below:

▸ Saturated fats are normally solid at room temperature and include the fats found in most animal products (meat, dairy products and eggs) and certain vegetable oils (e.g. coconut oil, palm and palm kernel oil, cocoa butter). Trans fats are oils that have been chemically altered through hydrogenation (or partial hydrogenation) to make them more saturated.

▸ Monounsaturated fats, found in foods such as olive oil, peanut oil, canola oil, olives, peanuts, nuts and avocados, tend to lower total blood cholesterol. Especially significant is their tendency to lower the damaging form of cholesterol contained in Low Density Lipoproteins (LDL) while preserving the so-called "good" cholesterol contained in High Density Lipoproteins (HDL). HDLs carry cholesterol from the coronary arteries back to the liver where it is broken down. (Regular exercise is the best way to increase HDL levels in the body.)

▸ Polyunsaturated fats are also known to lower cholesterol and include such common oils as corn, safflower, soybean and sunflower seed. Omega-3 fatty acids are a unique type of polyunsaturated fat that show promise in preventing heart disease. Flaxseed oil, walnuts and fatty fish (particularly the cold water varieties such as mackerel, salmon, sardines and tuna) are rich in omega-3 fatty acids.

▸ Cholesterol is a waxy fatlike substance produced by the body and consumed in the diet. Blood cholesterol levels vary between individuals and are influenced by both genetics and diet. Dietary cholesterol is found only in animal foods. Full-fat dairy products, egg yolks, animal fat and liver are the most common sources of dietary cholesterol.

▲ Guidelines from the National Cholesterol Education Program recommend that children over the age of two average no more than 30 percent of their total calories from fat, 10 percent or fewer of their calories from saturated fat and limit cholesterol to no more than 300 milligrams each day. The guidelines also advocate that children eat a wide variety of foods and consume enough calories to support growth and development.

▲ Not every single food eaten has to meet the guideline for 30 percent fat calories. It is the balance of the entire daily (or even weekly) diet that should register 30 percent or fewer fat calories. (See Chapter 6 for information on calculating calories from fat.)

⌗ PULSE RATE

Teach children to monitor their pulse rates using their index and middle fingers on either the wrist or neck (carotid pulse). An easy way to find the carotid pulse is to place the thumb of the right hand on the chin and then search with the first two fingers until the pulse feels strong and steady. Time the pulse for six seconds, instructing children when to start and stop counting. Multiply the number times 10 for the beats-per-minute pulse rate.

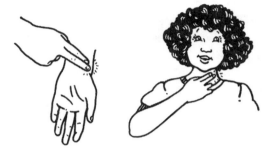

ACTIVITIES

▲ Contrast resting heart rate with active heart rate. (The resting heart rate for an average child is around 80 beats per minute.) Have children take their pulse at rest and record. Next, have them jump rope or run in place for 1–2 minutes, checking pulse immediately after they finish. What happens to the pulse rate?

▲ Ask students to keep a pulse rate chart, noting how their heart rate responds to different situations, such as waking up, after eating, when scared or nervous, before bed, during active play or exercise, etc.

▲ Assign students math problems that use their pulse data. For instance, using resting pulse rate, calculate how many times the heart

> Laqueesha's
> Pulse Rate
> When I wake up 73
> At a scary movie 94
> After riding my bike 120
> Doing Homework 82

beats each day, week, month, etc. How many extra beats does 30 minutes of exercise or active play add to the total each day? Does the resting pulse rate vary between children in the class? Are there differences between girls and boys? Plot the results in a table or show graphically.

▲ Pose the following "challenge question" to students: Will a heart made strong through regular exercise beat faster or slower when at rest? (Answer: The resting heart rate is slower because a strong heart can pump more blood with fewer beats. Many endurance athletes have resting pulse rates as low as 40 beats per minute.)

▲ Target pulse rate is the heart rate to strive for during an aerobic work-out such as running, jumping rope, swimming, biking or skating. To build a strong heart, it is recommended that children exercise at their target pulse rates (shown in Table 11-2) a minimum of 20 continuous minutes, three times weekly.

Table 11-2

TARGET PULSE RATE

Resting Rate	Target Rate
below 60	150
60–64	152
65–69	153
70–74	154
75–79	155
80–84	158
85–89	161
90 & above	163

Source: Learning91, July/August 1991, by Bruce Fisher, Chris Hopper, and Kathy Munoz

EATING FOR A HEALTHY HEART

Discuss how *MyPyramid* can be a helpful tool in planning a heart-healthy diet. Ask children to list choices from each food group that contribute to good heart health. Discuss how some choices in the dairy and protein group vary greatly in their cholesterol and saturated fat content. For instance, contrast the fat content of skinless baked chicken and fried chicken, whole and 1% milk, ground beef and dried beans or fat-free yogurt and cheese.

ACTIVITIES

▲ Using the blank *MyPyramid* on page 52, have students design their version of a heart-healthy *MyPyramid*.

▲ Ask students why they think *Nutrition Facts* food labels contain information on saturated fat and trans fat. (ANSWER: Saturated and trans fat have the most direct link to high blood cholesterol level.) Visit a grocery store or bring in a variety of food labels and compare saturated and trans fat contents. Examples include butter and margarine (see Chapter 6, page 92), different types of milk, a variety of cheeses, labels from meat products and snack items such as cookies and crackers.

YOU WILL NEED:

- Label information from a variety of foods (see text)

▲ **How Fat Clogs Arteries** Utilize the classroom water table or rubber basins to emulate the process of how fat affects arteries. You will need clear plastic tubing, solid vegetable shortening, cotton swabs and red food coloring. Fill the water table or basin with water; add red food coloring. Explain to the students that the water represents blood, the tubes are arteries and the shortening is fat that deposits in the arteries. Children can play and experiment, noting how a dab of fat in the tubing impairs "blood flow," and what happens when the tubing is totally blocked with fat. (Remind children that the process of fat accumulation in the arteries takes many years and is not the result of an occasional fatty meal.)

YOU WILL NEED:

- Clear, flexible tubing

- Solid vegetable shortening

- Cotton swabs

- Red food coloring

- Water table or rubber basin

Goal Setting

When making any kind of habit change, it's important to set a goal and keep track of progress. This is especially true for health behaviors, since they involve changing daily habits. Children, especially those younger than age 12, have a definite advantage since their lifetime habits are still under construction.

ACTIVITY

▲ Encourage children to set weekly health, nutrition or fitness goals. It is important to record progress toward the goal, which can be as simple as a checkmark on a chart, a daily bar to color on a graph or a simple entry in a health journal. Consider individual as well as classroom goals.

Examples of individual goals might be to participate in active play after school at least 20 minutes, four days a week or choose a healthful after-school snack each day. Classroom goals might consist of five minutes of daily relaxation or a minimum of two 20-minute classroom walks each week.

Goals should be simple, achievable and easy to measure. It is also important to reward achieved goals. Nonfood rewards are best and can range from classroom privileges, stickers, bookmarks and pencils to business-donated items such as movie passes, water bottles or gift certificates.

Eating for Exercise

THE BEST FUEL

Active kids do best when they fuel their bodies with a high-energy diet. During exercise, carbohydrate fuels the hard-working muscles via break-down of **glycogen**, the storage form of carbohydrate that releases glucose during muscle work. The body also relies on a steady stream of blood glucose to fuel all body systems, even the brain.

The best way to replenish the body's carbohydrate stores is to eat a diet rich in grains, beans, fruits and vegetables. The more active the child, the more carbohydrate is needed for refueling. Fatigue, "burn out" and lack of stamina can all be signs that body carbohydrate stores are low.

ACTIVITY

Create analogies between the active body and an automobile. Have the children expand and explain the similarities, using the following examples: Gasoline is to a car like (food) is to a body; a body that runs out of carbohydrate is like a car that runs out of (gasoline); filling a car with high-octane fuel is like feeding the athlete with a high-(carbohydrate) diet; an engine is fueled by gasoline in the same way the working (muscles) are fueled by carbohydrates.

Encourage children to write and illustrate stories that show the analogy between fueling a car and feeding a body.

THE MOST IMPORTANT NUTRIENT

Water is actually the nutrient of most immediate concern to the young athlete. During training or competition, thirst is not a good indicator of fluid needs. Not only will dehydration impair a child's performance, it also poses a severe, immediate health risk. Frequent water breaks, especially in warm weather, are a necessity. Each pound of water lost through sweat should be replaced with 16 ounces (2 cups) of fluid.

Kids should be encouraged to drink before, during and after practice and events. Plain water is the best choice, since it is cheap and readily available. Sports drinks, with their relatively low sugar concentration, make suitable fluid replacements as well. Pop, juice and other high-sugar beverages are not good choices because they slow the absorption of water from the stomach into the body.

ACTIVITIES

Weigh children prior to an active physical education class, a sporting event or other physical activity, and again afterward. Have each child calculate how much weight was lost. Explain that the weight change was due to water loss from perspiration. Ask children to calculate how much fluid they should drink to replace the loss. (For more accurate results, instruct children to use the restroom before weighing and monitor fluids consumed during the activity.)

▲ Have students keep a record of fluid intake throughout the day. Include water, juice, milk and soft drinks as well as less obvious sources such as frozen treats, soup and other liquid foods. A minimum of eight cups of fluid each day is recommended and the active child will need even more. Suggest students set goals related to their daily fluid intake.

During the busy school day, children often forget to drink fluids. Remind students to drink water at recess, before or after breaks and at lunchtime.

PRE-EVENT EATING

What and when a young athlete eats can influence the outcome of practice or the big game. The hard-working muscles should be well fueled for activity. This is accomplished with a meal that is eaten two to three hours prior to the start of an event. On practice days, a snack or light meal can be eaten up to one hour before.

It is best to have the stomach as empty as possible during physical activity. Normally, blood is diverted to the vessels surrounding the digestive tract right after eating. Likewise, physical activity requires a lion's share of the blood to supply exercising muscles with fuel and oxygen. Exercising with food in the stomach stages a competition between the muscles and digestive tract, resulting in poor physical performance as well as an upset stomach.

Foods high in complex carbohydrates, moderate in protein and low in fat and sugar are ideal for pre-exercise meals. The energy in sugar is short-lived while greasy foods hang in the stomach for hours (see Chapter 7, page 105, for an explanation of fat digestion). Fluids should also be emphasized prior to physical activity.

Good nutrition is also important after the game. This is the time to replenish the body's stores of carbohydrate and other key nutrients with a healthful, balanced meal.

ACTIVITIES

▲ On the board or overhead, stage a "digestion race," where students determine which foods they think will take longer to leave their stomachs. Pair foods with identical serving sizes, but varying amounts of fat. Examples include pretzels versus potato chips, a bagel versus a doughnut, high-fat versus low-fat crackers or ice cream versus frozen yogurt.

Ask students to explain the differences between the two foods, noting which will take longer to digest and why. Share *Nutrition Facts* label information from the products with the students, asking them to note the fat content of the two foods. Discuss which food is better to eat prior to exercise.

YOU WILL NEED:

- Label information for foods used in this activity

▲ Assign students the task of planning a precompetition meal. Meals must be high in carbohydrate, moderate in protein, low in fat and paired with a beverage. Students can get ideas from the sample meals listed in Table 11-3.

Table 11-3

PRE-EXERCISE MEALS

The simple-to-fix meals below are great before practice or games or as light meals between events during an all-day competition. Pair them with a piece of fruit and low-fat milk or water.

- Pita bread stuffed with tuna salad (made with light mayonnaise), tomato slice and sprouts
- Bagel sandwich made of lean turkey, lettuce leaf and a dab of light mayonnaise
- English muffin split and topped with pizza sauce, vegetables and mozzarella cheese; broiled until melted
- Pretzels or pretzel chips and string cheese
- Peanut butter & fruit sandwich on whole-wheat bread (try applesauce, sliced banana or raisins)
- Baked potato topped with reduced-fat or fat-free salad dressing
- Tortilla stuffed with hot refried beans, a sprinkle of cheese, shredded lettuce, diced tomato and salsa
- Pasta with marinara sauce, a sprinkle of parmesan cheese and baby carrots

Suggest that students interview a local athlete about his or her diet. The student should find out what the athlete typically eats in a day, favorite foods, meals eaten before competition, foods the athlete avoids and any special food or nutrition habits that help the athlete to perform better. Ask the student to write a report and/or present the information to the class. (But keep in mind that sometimes even the best athletes don't always practice good nutrition!)

Food Games

Active games that promote nutrition concepts can be creative and fun. The following games reinforce the principles of *MyPyramid* as students engage in active play. Encourage children to develop their own games that center on a food or nutrition theme.

ACTIVITIES

▲ **Let's Make a Meal Relay** Reproduce the food group cards on page 182, cut them out and place them in a hat. Be sure to include several copies of each food group (grains, vegetables, fruits, milk, and meat & beans.) Have each student draw a card from the hat. The objective is for students to form a relay team made up of five members, with each student on the team representing a different food group.

Explain that when you blow your whistle (or yell "Go"), students are to mingle, share with classmates which food group they represent and organize into "complete meal" teams. (Warning: This is a noisy game!) Once a team is assembled, each team member will run an assigned length, relay style. The first team to finish is the winner.

▲ **Build a *MyPyramid* Scramble** Similar to the meal relay, students will again draw food group slips out of a hat. The objective is for the students to scramble and organize themselves in the formation of *MyPyramid* as quickly as possible. Refer to the inside back cover for placement of the food groups in *MyPyramid*. Use a stopwatch to time students, noting their improvement with subsequent efforts.

▲ **Jump Rope Jingles** Ask students to invent jingles with a nutrition twist. For example, "Eating *MyPyramid* at my dinner, name each group and be the winner," followed by the child calling out a different food group for each jump (e.g., rice/jump, carrots/jump, peach/jump, chicken/jump, milk/jump). The goal is to name a food from a different food group with every jump. (It's harder than it first appears!)

Encourage students to put a new twist on old favorites. For example, "Cinderella dressed in teal; Went inside to eat her meal; How many _____ (insert food group name here) did she eat?" Call out the names of foods that are in the selected food group with a different food corresponding to each jump.

FOOD GROUP CARDS

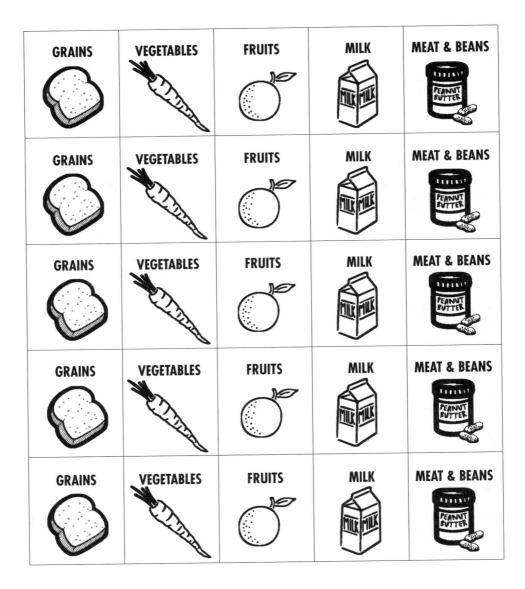

Reproduce, cut apart, and use in food group games

The Walking Classroom

According to Carolyn Johnson, a Portland, Oregon, elementary teacher, "just about anything you teach in the classroom can be done on a walk."

Carolyn, a serious walker herself, "takes her classroom beyond four walls" by integrating walking into all areas of her curriculum. She divides walking into three categories: fitness walking, "taking a break" walking and walking field trips and games.

FITNESS WALKING

When Carolyn takes her class on a fitness walk, she emphasizes a pace that is consistent, steady and relatively uninterrupted. She works on warming up, cooling down, stretching, appropriate pacing and

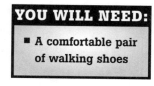

YOU WILL NEED:
- A comfortable pair of walking shoes

good posture with her students. During fitness walks, she exposes her class to different walking paces and varying terrain.

On soggy Oregon days that are too wet for an outside walk, Carolyn sets up a classroom fitness circuit.

TAKE A BREAK

Carolyn takes her class on short walks as a type of mental break. "Studies show that short walks can give us an energy boost and help to improve our mood," states Johnson. She gives her class walking breaks before an assembly when quiet sitting will be expected, when they need a "breather" and when they have been working hard and need a change of pace. She also walks with her class the first few minutes of each recess.

DISCOVERY WALKS

Carolyn incorporates academics into walking by taking discovery field trips around the school neighborhood. Her students become meteorologists by observing, graphing and measuring weather; monitoring the evaporation rates of puddles and creating big books based on their findings. They watch trees change throughout the seasons; note different colors, shapes and sounds and observe different forms of transportation. After a visit to a farm, her class walks to a neighborhood grocery store to see where the harvested food goes (and later develop a classroom grocery store based on their newfound knowledge).

Carolyn naturally incorporates her teaching of nutrition and healthful lifestyle habits into her classroom walks. "Perhaps the greatest reward from our daily walks is the growth of each child's self-esteem. Everyone is successful at walking and everyone has fun."

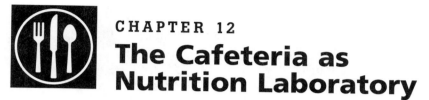

CHAPTER 12

The Cafeteria as Nutrition Laboratory

"I'm looking forward to coming and seeing the central kitchen. I like the food that your factory cooks." —Jonathan

As the nutrition lesson I was presenting came to a close, one of the first graders invited me to stay and eat lunch with her. Soon, several more children chimed in, pleading for me to be their guest in the school cafeteria. Curious to experience school lunch from a new perspective, I agreed.

As we crowded together to eat, I felt surrounded by adults giving directions over a microphone, pacing up and down the aisles and hurrying each table off to play. My "classmates" warned me not to talk too much or too loudly. Before I had eaten half my meal, the cafeteria monitor excused our entire table! An eye-opening experience, lunch that day was a powerful reminder of how adult order and rules can sometimes bypass the needs of children.

Lunch is much more than a routine break in the middle of the school day. The cafeteria, at its best, *can* be an integral part of the education of students — offering children firsthand experience with nutritious food choices, a chance to socialize with friends and a pleasant atmosphere to recharge body and mind.

This visionary cafeteria is possible but requires time, effort and education to succeed. Training for nutrition staff, a commitment from school faculty and administration and support from parents and the community all contribute to a successful school meal program.

Presented here are ideas on how every school cafeteria can become a center for nutrition education. Of primary importance is a menu that features choices consistent with the *Dietary Guidelines for Americans.* Students entering the cafeteria can then easily recognize *MyPyramid* in action. This chapter also provides suggestions on how to enhance mealtime atmosphere and successfully market the school meal program.

For those worried about skin-tight budgets, the ideas outlined in this chapter make good business sense, too. A solid nutrition program — marketed right — increases participation and boosts image. A number of school cafeterias throughout the country have successfully advanced their programs by making health-minded changes.

School Meals: Part of a Healthful School Environment

One goal of *Healthy People 2010*, the set of federal objectives for health promotion, is "to increase the proportion of children and adolescents, aged 6 to 19, whose intake of meals and snacks at school contributes proportionally to good overall dietary quality."

Are we making progress toward this objective? The good news is that school meals have improved nutritionally over the past 10 years. The School Nutrition Dietary Assessment-II, released in early 2001, shows big improvements over the same study conducted in 1992. Fat levels in school meals have dropped significantly, and a majority of school districts have increased the number of fruit, vegetable and grain choices offered in school lunches.

But unfortunately, while USDA-sponsored school meals have improved, the overall school environment for healthful eating has declined. The reason is primarily due to the large influx of "competitive foods," (i.e., foods offered at schools that are not part of the USDA school meal programs). Examples include food items sold from vending machines, student stores, after-school fundraisers and a la carte sales in the cafeteria. While it is possible to serve healthful choices from these venues, the reality is that most of the competitive foods marketed to children are of low nutritional quality.

Non-USDA foods sold in schools affect the daily dietary intakes of school-age children, according to a 2001 report presented to Congress by the USDA. Based on the report, very few school-age children meet the USDA's *Dietary Guidelines*, and therefore their intakes of nutrients such as calcium, phosphorous and vitamin A are lower than they should be.

The authors of the report maintain that competitive foods 1) have diet-related health risks because they lack the nutrients necessary for growth and learning; 2) may stigmatize school meal programs as being only for children with low incomes; 3) may affect the viability of school meal programs because of declining participation and 4) result in children receiving a mixed message, because while they are learning about good nutrition in the classroom they are presented with low-nutrient-density food options outside the classroom.

WHAT SCHOOLS CAN DO

Ultimately, it's up to each individual school to make significant progress toward a healthful school environment, promoting healthful school food services as well as the goals pertaining to school health and physical education.

For starters, score your program using the self-assessment checklist in Table 12-1. This "checklist for success" is a quick, helpful tool in evaluating your program and setting goals for improvement. For a more comprehensive assessment of your school's health environment, you may want to administer the *School Health Index for Physical Activity and Healthy Eating*, a comprehensive tool from the Centers for Disease Control and Prevention. You can access the School Health Index at *www.cdc.gov/nccdphp/dash/SHI*.

The remainder of this chapter is devoted to providing practical, hands-on ideas for improving the school nutrition environment on a local level.

Table 12-1

HEALTHFUL SCHOOL ENVIRONMENT: CHECKLIST FOR SUCCESS

Are you making the grade when it comes to a healthful school nutrition environment? Rate your efforts and see for yourself!

_____ 1. Do your menus meet the nutrition standards of the *Dietary Guidelines for Americans* and *MyPyramid*? (3=absolutely; 2=they could use some improvement; 1=not really)

_____ 2. Do your menus take into consideration student preferences and offer a variety of choices that appeal to various ethnic groups in your school? (3=absolutely; 2=they could use some improvement; 1=not really)

_____ 3. Do you offer students a positive eating environment with adequate time to eat? (3=yes, at a majority of schools in the district; 2=at some schools; 1=not really)

_____ 4. Does your school or district have a coordinated school nutrition policy that promotes healthful eating? (3=yes; 2=it's in development; 1=no)

_____ 5. Is there a comprehensive nutrition education curriculum in place in your district? (3=yes; 2=it's in development; 1=no)

_____ 6. Is the school foodservice department integrated with classroom nutrition education? (3=yes, we work on several programs and activities; 2=somewhat, on occasion at some schools; 1=no)

_____ 7. Is there a competitive food policy in place that prohibits the direct competition of minimally nutritious foods with the school meal program? (3=yes; 2=it's in development; 1=no)

_____ 8. Do you provide your staff with ongoing inservice training in nutrition and personal wellness? (3=yes; 2=only occasionally; 1=no)

_____ 9. Are family members and the community involved in supporting and reinforcing nutrition education? Do you reach out to parents and other adults with your nutrition education efforts? (3=yes, frequently; 2=only occasionally; 1=rarely)

_____ 10. Do you have an evaluation component in place to measure your progress in reaching nutrition education goals? (3=yes, for all our efforts; 2=only on some programs; 1=no)

How did you do? If you got a perfect score of 30, congratulations! I hope you are sharing your ideas and success stories with colleagues from other districts. If you scored 15 or higher, you are making progress. Keep up the good work and don't get discouraged. If you scored below 15, don't despair! Start by taking just one or two categories and really concentrating your efforts in these areas over the next year.

Source: Evers C. A nutrition education report card. School Foodservice & Nutrition. June/July 2000.

Nutrition in the Cafeteria

IMPLEMENTING THE DIETARY GUIDELINES

Using the *Dietary Guidelines for Americans* to plan and prepare school meals is not difficult, especially if changes are made gradually. Involving students in the process is more likely to result in a successful transition (see "Ask the Students" section below).

Technical assistance is available to programs seeking healthful changes. Child Nutrition personnel at the state level can often serve as technical consultants and trainers for schools implementing a healthful menu and nutrition education program. Appendix B lists organizations that provide school foodservice professionals with menus, recipes and other resources useful in implementing the dietary guidelines.

School meal programs throughout the country are as diverse and varied as the individuals they serve. But in spite of cultural, geographic and ethnic differences, all schools can succeed at making the cafeteria a healthful environment. Table 12-2 lists easy-to-implement changes that make a big nutritional difference in the menu.

OFFER CHOICE & VARIETY

From clothing to entertainment to careers, today's children have a multitude of choices compared to previous generations. The same is true for food — children definitely want a say in what they eat.

Schools can devise a system of variety and choice that improves nutrition habits and reduces waste. A number of school districts have successfully implemented this type of system at the elementary level, offering a choice of three or more entrées and self-serve variety bars which feature a wide selection of fruits, vegetables and breads.

Table 12-2

15 STEPS TOWARD MEETING THE
DIETARY GUIDELINES

1. Use fat-free yogurt as the base for fruit and vegetable dips, salad dressings, tartar sauce and breakfast toppings. Besides lowering the fat in these products, yogurt adds calcium, protein and other nutrients.

2. Substitute reduced-fat mayonnaise for the full-fat variety. The reduced variety tastes nearly the same and contains about half the fat as regular mayo.

3. Increase the fiber in baked products by using whole-wheat flour. If acceptance is a problem, begin by using a small amount in a recipe (25 percent), gradually increasing the ratio of whole-wheat to white flour. Another way to boost fiber and nutrients is to add wheat germ, bran or bulgur to baked goods.

4. Always have several fruit and vegetable choices available. Purchase canned fruits packed in water or fruit juice. When cooking vegetables, lightly steam to preserve quality and nutrients.

5. Experiment with lower-fat cheeses. Part-skim mozzarella is well accepted and can be used on pizza, in Mexican dishes and sliced for sandwiches. Test different varieties of reduced-fat cheddar and American to find brands that are acceptable in taste and texture.

6. Reduce the amount of butter used in cooking. Vegetables and rolls don't need to be slathered with gobs of butter. If possible, switch to a soft margarine product that is free of trans fat.

7. When serving pizza, always offer at least one vegetarian choice. Experiment with new vegetable combinations such as pepper rings, broccoli florets, shredded carrots or chopped spinach. Layer vegetables on top of sauce, then cover with cheese — a sneaky way to get kids to eat their vegetables!

8. Use the leanest ground meat available, whether lean beef or turkey. Always drain after browning (rinsing with hot water removes even more fat without loss of quality).

9. Plant flowers in the deep fryer! Prepare most foods by oven baking, broiling or steaming.

10. Limit the choice of hot dogs and corn dogs — high in both fat and salt — to no more than once a month.

Table 12-2 (continued)

11. Merchandise low-fat milk (1% or lower) as the milk of choice (although other milks can still be offered).

12. Remove salt shakers from lunchroom tables.

13. Offer nutritious breakfast items that are low in sugar, such as English muffins, whole grain bagels, low-sugar cold cereals and whole-wheat toast. Reserve high-sugar muffins, sweet rolls and doughnuts as occasional choices. Purchase reduced-sugar syrup for pancakes, French toast and waffles. Other nutritious breakfast choices include yogurt, fresh fruit and leftover pizza or sandwiches.

14. Write purchasing specifications with nutrition in mind. Clearly state the upper limits of fat, sodium, sugar, etc. that you define as acceptable in a particular product. Insist that nutritionally modified products meet taste and quality standards.

15. Work with manufacturers to develop and offer nutritious products that are acceptable to children. Offer to test and evaluate new items in your program.

One Oregon school (North Plains Elementary) witnessed particularly dramatic changes after the implementation of the choice system. Average daily lunch participation increased from 61 percent to 73 percent, the produce order jumped from 40 to 100 pounds per week and the amount of food left uneaten on the average tray dropped 47 percent. By keeping an eye on the garbage cans and adjusting production accordingly, the school actually saw the average food cost per meal drop 16 percent. Because students were selecting much of their lunches, serving time was ultimately reduced (once children got the "hang" of it) and labor costs held steady.

A cafeteria that features variety and choice also provides options for children who are vegetarian, have specific ethnic preferences or have medical conditions such as diabetes, food allergies or lactose intolerance.

Guidelines for implementing this type of system are included in Table 12-3.

Table 12-3

TIPS FOR IMPLEMENTING A SELF-SERVE MENU CHOICE SYSTEM

The students in Oregon's *"Food Pyramid Choice Menu"* elementary schools are given a lunchtime selection of three or more healthful entrées, a choice of milks and a self-serve variety bar loaded with fruits, vegetables and bread/grain items. The following guidelines will help you get started in setting up a similar system.

▲ Obtain school board approval before introducing this new style of meal service in elementary or middle school cafeterias.

▲ Plan the physical design of the new system. Evaluate and order equipment and supplies as needed (e.g., self-serve bars matched to student height, bread baskets, trays, tongs, etc.). Make sure the cafeteria layout includes space for an adult to monitor trays at the **end** of the service area.

▲ Offer a variety of nutritious choices of all food components. Consider offering standard choices along with rotating choices each day. Fresh fruits and vegetables are generally more popular than the cooked or canned varieties.

▲ Education is central to the success of this program! Nutrition staff, teachers and administrators should be well prepared to explain the rationale and procedure of the new system to students. Parents should receive written information detailing the new program, including an invitation to eat lunch with their children (Consider hosting a "grand opening" to highlight the program two to three weeks after its inception.)

▲ Be prepared for challenges and possibly extra labor in the first few days. Stock up on extra fruits, vegetables, breads and other "variety bar" items.

▲ Integrate the cafeteria changes into classroom education. Highlight how this program positively impacts nutrition, meets the needs of more students and how the reduction in food waste is good for the environment.

The guidelines in this table are adapted from a report prepared by Harding Lawson Associates (HLA), a private environmental engineering firm that conducted waste prevention pilot projects at three Oregon elementary schools.

ASK THE STUDENTS!

When making menu changes, the best "consultants" you can obtain are free and readily available — they are the students you serve each day.

When kids feel ownership in the meal program, they are more likely to support and patronize school breakfast and lunch. Revamping the menu without the students' knowledge or support can drive students away from the school meal program.

Since food becomes nutrition only after it is eaten, menu changes should reflect students' food preferences. One way to elicit this information is to form student advisory groups. Some schools refer to these as Nutrition Advisory Councils (NACs).

Education is the key to making advisory councils work effectively. Students should first gain a clear understanding of the goals of the school meal program, which is to provide a variety of nutritious foods that students will eat and to operate the program in a cost-effective manner. Ideally, students selected for the council will have some basic understanding of nutrition and why it is important. If not, this may be an ideal forum for hands-on nutrition education activities.

Children can also gain skills in constructive criticism and problem solving. Some students may be reluctant to offer feedback, while others may present a very negative picture of the school cafeteria (we've all heard the jokes and negative comments). A sample dialogue that I have used successfully with students is included in Table 12-4.

Role of the Advisory Council The advisory council can participate in the school meal program in a variety of ways. Examples of NAC activities are outlined below.

▲ Poll the student body to find out the most- and least-liked favorite foods served at school. Brainstorm ways that favorite foods can be modified to meet the *Dietary Guidelines for Americans*.

▲ Conduct plate waste studies to determine which foods are consistently thrown out, uneaten (see Chapter 7, page 116 for an example).

Table 12-4

TEACHING CONSTRUCTIVE CRITICISM

Students, particularly those in the intermediate grades, may resort to negative remarks when describing the food served at school. Responding to students in a defensive and critical manner only serves to worsen the situation. Below is a sample dialogue that illustrates how to defuse the situation and promote cooperative problem solving.

LEADER: Would anyone like to share their thoughts about the school breakfast or lunch program?

STUDENT 1: It's so-o-o-o-o gross!

STUDENT 2: Yeah, I wouldn't feed that nasty junk to my dog!

LEADER: What I think I'm hearing is that some of you dislike the food served in the cafeteria. The problem is, I haven't heard much useful information so far. Right now, if I were to sit down and plan next month's menu, the comments I just heard sure wouldn't help me much.

STUDENT 3: I have a complaint — sometimes when I eat the third lunch period, the milk has been sitting out for a while and it's warm.

LEADER: Thank you. It helps when you give me a specific example of a problem that you see in the cafeteria. You have a valid point — milk should not sit at room temperature for that length of time. Do any of you have suggestions on how to solve this problem?

STUDENT 4: Maybe you could keep cartons of milk in a bowl filled with ice.

STUDENT 5: How about using one of those refrigerators that can be rolled into the cafeteria at lunchtime?

LEADER: Those are great suggestions, students. In fact, I'm going to start a list of your ideas that I can use in my planning.

STUDENT 1: Do you think you could do something so that the broccoli isn't mushy? My mom always serves it raw with ranch dip. I like it that way.

STUDENT 2: And I wish we could have a salad bar more often. I always eat lunch the days we have a salad bar.

LEADER: Thank you, students. It is very helpful when you give specific examples and useful suggestions. With your help, I can make changes that improve the program for everyone.

▲ Taste test and evaluate new recipes, commodities or vendor food items that have been nutritionally "improved" (e.g., reduced in fat, salt or sugar, whole-wheat flour substituted for white, fortified with calcium, etc.).

▲ Plan a menu once a month, designating it as "NAC" day. To give students real-world experience, teach them to cost out the menu and perform a nutritional analysis of their chosen meal, making adjustments as needed.

▲ Train advisory council members as peer educators. Provide them with simple lesson ideas that they can teach in classrooms around the school. Suggest they develop and perform a noontime skit on good nutrition for the student body (see Chapter 9 for ideas).

▲ Enlist the advisory council's help in devising a marketing plan. Involve members in the development of a cafeteria slogan, logo, mascot or catchy name.

▲ Give the advisory council space on the menu for a "student's corner" where they can provide tips about nutrition and facts about the school meal program.

▲ Be sure to acknowledge and reward the work of the advisory council. Award students with special privileges, certificates or prizes such as pencils, notepads, stickers, water bottles or movie coupons.

COMPETITIVE FOODS — TAKING A STAND

The availability of competitive food, (i.e., foods with low nutrient density that are available for sale during the school day), undermines nutrition and health goals. When children can choose between a candy bar from the school store or a healthful lunch in the cafeteria, too often the candy bar will win out.

The issue of competitive foods is complex, often evoking debate among school foodservice providers, administrators and even parent groups. In times of stretched budgets, school groups, athletic teams and administrators resort to the sale of candy, pop, fried chips, cookies and other low-nutrition foods — often through vending machines — to boost revenues.

While some states and school districts have official policies banning or restricting competitive foods, many schools choose to ignore the issue, fearful of "rocking the boat."

Unpopular as the issue may be, it is important to highlight the competitive food issue in each school. Offering healthful alternatives for fundraisers, stocking vending machines with more nutritious food and beverage choices and limiting student store sales to nutritious foods are all positive steps to creating a more healthful school environment.

At the very least, a compromise should be agreed on and enforced that limits the sale of foods with low nutrient density to after school or during sporting events.

Cafeteria Atmosphere

FROM DRAB TO DELIGHTFUL

With effort and creativity, the school cafeteria can become a bright and cheery place to eat. Some ideas:

▲ Paint can do wonders for the cafeteria. Replace drab, boring walls with blocks of bright colors. Or invite the art teacher or a guest artist to coordinate students in the design and painting of a colorful cafeteria mural. (A food and fitness theme would be especially nice!)

▲ Collect and frame colorful posters of food to display them near the serving areas. (Many of the food companies listed in Appendix B provide free posters and other materials for display.)

▲ Encourage students to design posters that depict good nutrition themes for the cafeteria.

▲ Display a "nutrition corner" bulletin board that is changed regularly throughout the year. Examples of themes include *MyPyramid*, food and fitness, how food promotes a healthy heart, how to read the *Nutrition Facts* food label, the importance of calcium in building strong bones, how breakfast fuels learning and facts about the school meal program. Consider a nearby table with handout information for students, staff and parents. Teachers, students and school foodservice staff can work cooperatively to design and maintain the bulletin board throughout the year.

▲ Add a personal touch to the cafeteria: Spruce up the serving line with colorful garnishes, display bright vinyl tablecloths on serving tables (fabric stores are an inexpensive source of colorful vinyl), purchase or make eye-catching aprons for nutrition staff and student assistants or occasionally put out fresh cut flowers on cafeteria tables.

TIME TO EAT

Offering tasty, nutritious food in a pleasant environment is not enough, though — children must have time to eat. It sounds simple enough, yet schools pressed for instructional time frequently shortchange kids by skimping on lunch time. Shortened lunch periods, coupled with long lines and slow service, may give children as few as five minutes to eat! In some schools, students opt for sack lunches just so they can bypass the lunch line.

From the time children sit down with their tray, they should be guaranteed a minimum of 20 uninterrupted minutes to eat. More time may be required for students with certain disabilities. The same holds true for breakfast — bus and morning schedules should be adjusted to allow ample time for children eating breakfast at school.

Marketing & Education

TOOT YOUR HORN!

Many school nutrition operators would do well to boast more, spreading the *good* news about their programs. Students, teachers and parents may not know, for instance, that the "chicken nuggets" printed on the menu are actually a low-fat product or that the dinner rolls contain 50 percent whole-wheat flour or that a fruit and vegetable bar is available daily. They may be unaware of point-of-choice nutrition information in the cafeteria or special promotions or classroom nutrition lessons taught by nutrition staff.

Effectively communicating your message is an essential ingredient to marketing success. The first step is to define your target markets. This could include the children you serve, school personnel (teachers, staff, administrators) or the community (parents, school board, media). Next, devise ways to reach these groups with your message. The examples below highlight techniques for publicizing the school meal program.

▲ Start with the menu. An already familiar piece, the menu adorns thousands of refrigerators each month throughout your school community. Reserve space on the *front* of the menu for nutrition tidbits, program highlights and announcements of special promotions. Use words that denote nutrition to describe foods offered on menus, such as "whole-grain" rolls, "low-fat" dressing, "garden fresh" broccoli florets or "oven-baked" chicken.

Think about the design of the menu, too. Avoid using the same standard format month after month. Use computer graphics to enhance the design of the menu or enlist the help of school staff (art teachers, district graphic artists and typesetters), if available.

▲ Become an integral part of the school environment. School foodservice staff should take a keen interest in the events and programs in their school. Participate in monthly staff meetings, contribute items to the school newsletter or volunteer to assist teachers with food and nutrition lesson planning.

▲ Be proactive by inviting parents, the school board or the media to eat school breakfast or lunch. Highlight the nutrition messages and healthful choices served each day in the cafeteria. Send out notices of special promotions, contests and events.

Don't let national press coverage about the downside of school meals mar your program. Prepare a fact sheet that highlights your mission, statistics about those you serve and a summary of positive outcomes. Send a press release to local media that emphasizes how your program offers healthful choices as well as nutrition education.

BECOME A PARTNER IN EDUCATION

The nutrition concepts taught in the classroom can effectively be reinforced in the cafeteria. Beyond a health-promoting menu, school foodservice providers can also participate in nutrition education through a variety of practices, activities and promotions:

Everyone in the kitchen is a Nutrition Educator!

Attention school nutrition staff! Have you ever:

▲ Nudged the fruit basket to the front of the counter so more students would be tempted to grab a piece?

▲ Put up eye-catching signage to promote a new healthful entrée?

▲ Greeted a student with, "See you at breakfast tomorrow"?

▲ Stocked the salad bar with fresh seasonal produce?

If you answered "yes" to any of the above, you are promoting good nutrition habits. Whether or not it's apparent, everyone who works in the school cafeteria also wears the title of nutrition educator.

▲ **Merchandise Healthful Foods** Make sure healthful food choices beg to be eaten. The use of baskets, attractive arrangements, colorful food choices and garnishes will make nutritious foods stand out.

▲ **Point-of-Choice Nutrition Information** Display a simple nutrition analysis of foods commonly served in the cafeteria. (Consider working with a fourth or fifth grade class on determining and displaying the information.)

Include the analysis for calories, fat, carbohydrate, protein, cholesterol and sodium. Especially meaningful are comparisons of different forms of the same food such as 1% versus 2% versus whole milk, or pepperoni versus mushroom pizza.

Consider highlighting other nutrients from time to time, complemented by informative posters, bulletin boards and handouts. Examples include iron, fiber, B vitamins or calcium.

▲ **100 Percent Participation** You can achieve complete participation — one classroom at a time, that is. Once a month, set up a "make your own lunch" bar in a chosen classroom. Students will learn basic food preparation skills as they assemble their own meals. Food bars that work particularly well include a setup for submarine or pita-pocket sandwiches, chef salads, French bread pizza topped with vegetables or healthful nachos (made from reduced-fat corn chips, various beans, lean ground beef or ground turkey, low-fat cheese, salsa, olives, tomatoes, peppers, onions and low-fat plain yogurt). Cover and label each student's lunch to be passed out when they come through the serving line. (Or, if you have time, coordinate the activity right before their scheduled lunch period.)

If possible, make a lunch date with each classroom in the school over the course of the year. Besides being a great opportunity for nutrition education, this activity is also a powerful way to market the school meal program to students.

▲ **Promotions and Events** Make the cafeteria a fun place to learn with special promotions and thematic menus. "New Food Days" or "Food of the Week" events can feature small incentives for students who select a new healthful food. Menu, recipe or poster contests, nutrition bingo cards and breakfast ticket raffles are all fun ways to teach nutrition and promote the school meal program.

Posters, suggested menus and other resources are available for specific events such as National School Lunch Week (available through the School Nutrition Association) or National Nutrition Month (sponsored by the American Dietetic Association). There are also a multitude of other special holidays and months, celebrating everything from grandparents to pickles to potatoes to heart health!

▲ **Teaching Students** Many of the suggested nutrition activities and lessons described in Chapters 4–11 could easily be presented by school food and nutrition professionals. Nearly every chapter includes lesson ideas that interface with the cafeteria (identified by the cafeteria icon).

Inviting classes to tour the school or central kitchen is a memorable way to introduce students to the school nutrition operation. To enhance the experience, combine the tour with a brief lesson on nutrition, give students the opportunity to plan a menu, set up a taste test for a new product or challenge students to find a food from each food group.

School nutrition staff can also assist in career education, highlighting the job requirements and tasks of jobs such as cook, baker, chef, truck driver, school nutrition director, registered dietitian or food technologist.

Appendix A

GUIDELINES FOR SAFE CLASSROOM COOKING

"I liked how you served the food with your gloves. My Mom asked if anyone touched the food."—Jenny

With so many hands busy at work, classroom cooking poses a challenge for keeping food sanitary and working conditions safe. When planning cooking projects, be sure to enlist the help of school staff or parent volunteers. The reminders below are essential for a safe, enjoyable cooking experience.

BEFORE YOU BEGIN

▲ Send a letter home to parents explaining that the class will periodically participate in cooking projects that enhance the curriculum. *Be sure to elicit information on food allergies or intolerances or any specific medical conditions that prohibit their children from eating certain foods!* Include permission slips for parents to sign and return.

▲ Call the local health department to find out how to become certified as a food handler. You may be required to take a course or pass a test before handling food in a public setting (local and state regulations vary).

▲ Be sure that all staff and volunteers who assist with classroom cooking have read and understand the guidelines presented here.

"Fight Bac" is a great resource for food safety education materials and resources. Download and order materials at *www.fightbac.org*.

PROPER HANDWASHING IS VITAL!

▲ Demonstrate to students the techniques for proper handwashing. Thoroughly scrub all surfaces of the hands and nails with soap, rinse with warm water and dry with clean paper towels.

▲ The factor most important in producing clean hands is time. Encourage students to scrub hands for the duration of the "A-B-C song" (about 20 seconds).

▲ If the restroom is used for handwashing prior to handling food, prop the door open. Otherwise, students will touch the bacteria-covered doorknob on their way out.

▲ Remind students to wash hands after using the restroom; touching their faces, hair or neighbor; blowing their noses or sneezing and after handling raw meat, chicken, eggs or fish.

Tie in the concept of handwashing with a science lesson about bacteria and viruses. One kit that is especially helpful is the *Glitterbug Handwash Education System*, which uses a UV light and special soap to reveal whether hands contain "germs" (similar to the way dental disclosing tablets reveal the presence of plaque). Glitterbug products are available through Brevis Corporation, 225 West 2855 South, Salt Lake City, UT, 84115; *www.brevis.com*.

Another useful activity is to culture various surfaces such as hands, tables or doorknobs and grow on a nutrient-rich medium in a petri dish. Once the experiment is completed, petri dishes should be rinsed with a bleach solution and disposed of properly.

PROVIDE A SANITARY WORK SURFACE FOR HANDLING FOOD

▲ Desks or tables should be cleared, cleaned and covered with clean butcher paper or a vinyl placemat or tablecloth. Cutting boards should be cleaned with hot, soapy water and a sanitizing solution such as diluted bleach. (To make the bleach solution, mix 1 tablespoon institutional-strength bleach or 2 tablespoons household bleach into one gallon of water.)

▲ Wash and sanitize all work surfaces, cutting boards and utensils after they have come into contact with raw meat, fish, poultry or eggs.

EMPHASIZE SAFETY WITH KNIVES AND EQUIPMENT

▲ Before allowing children to begin work on food projects, demonstrate the proper use of knives and equipment such as graters, cheese slicers and can openers. Advise students to always cut toward their tables or desks and away from their hands.

▲ Any equipment, even plastic serrated knives, toothpicks or wooden skewers, can be dangerous if handled improperly. Promptly remove students who are behaving in a reckless manner with tools or equipment.

▲ Always use two dry potholders when removing foods from the microwave or oven. Be sure to turn off the stove, oven, electric fry pan, etc. when you are done cooking. Avoid knocking hot pots off the stove by turning pot and pan handles inward.

ORGANIZING COOKING PROJECTS

▲ For projects that students will prepare individually at their desks, assign three or four adult volunteers and/or students to hand out food and utensils. Those passing out supplies should practice good hygiene and always wear clean plastic gloves.

▲ One way to efficiently run a classroom cooking project is to organize an assembly line. Using a long table, line up the ingredients for such items as bagel pizzas, rolled burritos, stuffed pita sandwiches or fruit-yogurt parfaits. If you utilize this method, make sure there is at least one adult at both the beginning and end of the line. Just before starting through the line, students should put on clean plastic gloves.

▲ Time your projects so that foods do not sit at room temperature for more than two hours. The "danger zone" for rapid bacterial growth is between 40 and 140 degrees Fahrenheit (i.e., room temperature). Pick up foods from the kitchen right before you begin the project and return leftovers upon completion. Do not allow students to save perishable foods to eat later in the day.

▲ Don't sample food products prepared with raw eggs. Even one tasty spoonful of cookie batter could harbor dangerous bacteria. Recipes that call for raw eggs, such as eggnog or homemade ice milk, should use an egg substitute that has been pasteurized.

Appendix B

SELECTED RESOURCES

NOTE: Some companies and organizations are listed under more than one heading.

Audiovisual/Education Resource Catalogs

The following companies feature a wide variety of resources including videotapes, books, posters, computer software and props.

FOODPLAY PRODUCTIONS
    221 Pine Street
    Florence, MA 01062
    1-800-FOODPLAY
    www.foodplay.com

HEALTH EDCO
    P.O. Box 21207
    Waco, TX 76702-1207
    1-800-299-3366
    www.healthedco.com

NASCO Nutrition Teaching Aids Catalog
    901 Janesville Avenue
    P.O. Box 901
    Fort Atkinson, WI 53538-0901
    1-800-558-9595
    www.nascofa.com

NATIONAL HEALTH VIDEO
    11312 Santa Monica Blvd. #5
    Los Angeles CA 90025
    1-800-543-6803
    www.nhv.com

NCES (Nutrition, Counseling and Education Services)
  1904 E. 123rd
  Olathe, KS 66061
  1-877-623-7266
  www.ncescatalog.com

NEAT Solutions for Healthy Children
  P.O. Box 2432
  Martinez, CA 94553
  1-888-577-NEAT
  www.neatsolutions.com

YUMMY DESIGNS
  P.O. Box 1851
  Walla Walla, WA. 99362
  1-888-749-8669
  www.yummydesigns.com

Books For Children

See index entry "Books, Children" for a list of all children's books referenced throughout this book (coded by reading level).

Cookbooks for Kids

Albyn CL, Webb LS. *The Multicultural Cookbook for Students.* Oryx Press, 1993.

Cook DF. *The Kids' Multicultural Cookbook: Food & Fun Around the World.* Williamson Publishing, 1995.

D'Amico J, Drummond KE. *The Healthy Body Cookbook: Over 50 Fun Activities and Delicious Recipes for Kids,* John Wiley, 1999.

Nissenberg S. *The Everything Kids' Cookbook.* Adams Media Co., 2002.

Nissenberg S. *The Healthy Start Kids' Cookbook : Fun and Healthful Recipes That Kids Can Make Themselves*. John Wiley, 1994.

Warner P. *Healthy Snacks for Kids*. Bristol Publishing Enterprises, 2003.

Williamson S, Williamson Z. *Kids Cook!: Fabulous Food for the Whole Family*. Williamson Publishing, 2003.

Winston M. *American Heart Association KIDS' Cookbook*. Times Books, 1993.

Fitness

Children and Weight: What Communities Can Do
    Center for Weight and Health, U.C. Berkeley
    University of California
    101 Giannini Hall #3100
    Berkeley, CA 94720-3100
    www.cnr.berkeley.edu/cwh/activities/child_weight2.shtml

Jennings DS, Steen SN. *Play Hard, Eat Right: A Parent's Guide to Sports Nutrition for Children*. John Wiley, 1995.

Physical Best: Lifetime Fitness Education
    American Alliance for Health, Physical Education, Recreation & Dance
    1900 Association Dr.
    Reston, VA 20191-1598
    www.aahperd.org/physicalBest

The President's Challenge
    The President's Council on Physical Fitness and Sports
    Department W
    200 Independence Ave., SW
    Room 738-H
    Washington, D.C. 20201-0004
    Phone: 202-690-9000
    fitness.gov/challenge/challenge.html

Food Companies/Commissions

Food companies and commissions are often a great source for low-cost posters, flyers, recipes and nutrition education curricula.

A WORD OF CAUTION: Please read all company-sponsored materials carefully before using with students. Some materials may read like an advertisement or contain biased information. Choose materials that present a balanced view of nutrition.

American Dry Bean Board
    8233 Old Courthouse Road, Suite 210
    Vienna, VA 22182
    703-556-9304
    www.americanbean.org

California Kiwi Fruit Commission
    9845 Horn Road, Suite 160
    Sacramento, CA 95827
    916-362-7490
    www.kiwifruit.org

California Strawberry Commission
    PO Box 269
    Watsonville, CA 95077
    831-724-1301
    www.calstrawberry.com

California Table Grape Commission
    392 W. Fallbrook, Suite 101
    Fresno, CA 93711
    559-447-8350
    www.tablegrape.com

Canned Food Alliance
    www.mealtime.org

Dole 5 A Day Program
   One Dole Drive
   Westlake Village, CA 91362
   818-879-6772
   www.dole5aday.com

Florida Department of Citrus
   PO Box 148
   Lakeland, FL 33802
   863-499-2500
   www.floridajuice.com

International Food Information Council (IFIC) Foundation
   1100 Connecticut Avenue, N.W.
   Suite 430
   Washington, DC 20036
   202-296-6540
   www.ific.org

National Dairy Council
   10255 West Higgins Road, Ste. 900
   Rosemont, IL 60018
   www.nationaldairycouncil.org

Oregon Dairy Council/Nutrition Education Services
   10505 SW Barbur Blvd
   Portland, OR 97219
   503-229-5033
   www.oregondairycouncil.org

Produce for Better Health Foundation
   5341 Limestone Road
   Wilmington, DE 19808
   302-235-2329
   www.5aday.com

Pear Bureau Northwest
> 4382 SE International Way, Suite A
> Milwaukie, OR 97222
> 503-652-9720
> *www.usapears.com*

The Peanut Institute
> P.O. Box 70157
> Albany, Georgia 31708
> 888-8PEANUT
> *www.peanut-institute.org*

United States Potato Board
> 5105 E 41st Ave.
> Denver, Colorado 80216
> *www.potatohelp.com*

Washington State Apple Commission
> 2900 Euclid Avenue
> Post Office Box 18
> Wenatchee, WA 98807
> 509-663-9600
> *www.bestapples.com*

Washington State Fruit Commission/Northwest Cherries
> 105 South 18th Street, Suite 205
> Yakima, Washington 98901
> 509-453-4837
> *www.nwcherries.com*

Wheat Foods Council
> 10841 S. Crossroads Dr., Suite 105
> Parker, CO 80138
> 303-840-8787
> *www.wheatfoods.org*

Food Models

NASCO Nutrition Teaching Aids Catalog
901 Janesville Avenue
P.O. Box 901
Fort Atkinson, WI 53538-0901
1-800-558-9595
www.nascofa.com

National Dairy Council
10255 West Higgins Road, Ste. 900
Rosemont, IL 60018
www.nationaldairycouncil.org

NCES (Nutrition, Counseling and Education Services)
1904 E. 123rd
Olathe, KS 66061
1-877-623-7266
www.ncescatalog.com

Gardening

Farm to School/School Gardens
Healthy School Meals Resource System
Food and Nutrition Information Center
National Agriculture Library
10301 Baltimore Blvd., Rm 105
Beltsville, MD 20705-2351
301-504-6366
schoolmeals.nal.usda.gov/Resource/farmtoschool.htm

Growing with Plants
   Washington State University
   Pierce County Cooperative Extension
   3049 S 36th Street, Suite 300
   Tacoma, WA 98409
   253-798-7180
   www.pierce.wsu.edu/Nutrition/GWP

Kids Gardening
   National Gardening Association
   1100 Dorset Street
   South Burlington, VT 05403
   800-538-7476
   www.kidsgardening.com

Life Lab Science Program
   1156 High Street
   Santa Cruz, CA 95064
   831-459-2001
   www.lifelab.org

Patten E, Lyons K. *Healthy foods from healthy soils*. Tilbury House
   Publishers, 2003.

Garnishing

*The following books include colorful photographs and helpful illustrations
on creating garnishes.*

Kros W. *Fun Foods: Clever Ideas for Garnishing & Decorating*. Sterling
   Publishing Co., 1990

Lynch FT. *Garnishing: A Feast for Your Eyes*. HP Books, 1987.

Rosen H. *Garnishing for the Beginner*. International Culinary Consultants,
   1996.

Rosen H. *How to Garnish*. International Culinary Consultants, 1998.

General Reference

Duyff RL. American Dietetic Association *Complete Food and Nutrition Guide,* 2nd Edition. John Wiley, 2002.

Swinney B. *Healthy Foods for Healthy Kids.* Meadowbrook, 1999.

Webb FS, Whitney EN. *Nutrition Concepts and Controversies.* Wadsworth Publishing, 2002.

MyPyramid

Center for Nutrition Policy and Promotion
 U.S. Department of Agriculture
 3101 Park Center Drive, Rm. 1034
 Alexandria, VA 22302-1594
 703-305-7600
 www.usda.gov/cnpp

MyPyramid posters
 Order posters at *teachfree.com or mypyramid.gov*

MyPyramid Stickers
 Washington State Dairy Council
 4201 - 198th St. S.W. Suite 102
 Lynnwood, WA 98036
 206-744-1616
 www.eatsmart.org

Kids Health
 Visit the website below for a kid-friendly description of *MyPyramid*:
 www.kidshealth.org/kid/nutrition/food/pyramid.html

Team Nutrition
 U.S. Department of Agriculture, Food and Nutrition Service
 3101 Park Center Drive, Room 632
 Alexandria, VA 22302
 703-305-1624
 www.fns.usda.gov/tn

Nutrition Facts Food Label

Food Labeling and Nutrition
>U.S. Food and Drug Administration
>Center for Food Safety and Applied Nutrition
>5100 Paint Branch Parkway (HFS-555)
>College Park, MD 20740
>888-723-3366
>*vm.cfsan.fda.gov/label.html*

Organizations

American Dietetic Association
>120 South Riverside Plaza, Suite 2000
>Chicago, IL 60606-6995
>800-877-1600
>*www.eatright.org*

American Heart Association
>National Center
>7272 Greenville Avenue
>Dallas, TX 75231
>800-242-8721
>*www.americanheart.org*

California Foundation for Agriculture in the Classroom
>2300 River Plaza Drive
>Sacramento, CA 95833-3293
>916-561-5625
>*www.cfaitc.org*

Center for Science in the Public Interest
>1875 Connecticut Ave. N.W., Suite 300
>Washington, D.C. 20009
>202-332-9110
>*www.cspinet.org*

Food and Nutrition Information Center
National Agriculture Library
10301 Baltimore Blvd., Rm 105
Beltsville, MD 20705-2351
301-504-6366
www.nal.usda.gov/fnic

World Hunger Year (WHY)
505 Eighth Ave., Suite 2100
New York, NY 10018-6582
212-629-8850
www.worldhungeryear.org

Puppetry

Buetter B. *Simple Puppets From Everyday Materials.* Sterling Publishing, 1996.

Feller R, Feller M. *Paper Masks and Puppets for Stories, Songs, and Plays.* The Arts Factory, 1989.

Rump N. *Puppets and Masks: Stagecraft and Storytelling.* Davis Publications, 1995.

School Foodservice

Healthy School Meals Resource System
Food and Nutrition Information Center
National Agriculture Library
10301 Baltimore Blvd., Rm 105
Beltsville, MD 20705-2351
301-504-6366
schoolmeals.nal.usda.gov

National Food Service Management Institute
  The University of Mississippi
  P.O. Drawer 188
  University, MS 38677-0188
  800-321-3054
  www.olemiss.edu/depts/nfsmi

School Health Index for Physical Activity and Healthy Eating
  Centers for Disease Control and Prevention
  1600 Clifton Rd.
  Atlanta, GA 30333
  800-311-3435
  www.cdc.gov/nccdphp/dash/SHI

School Nutrition Association
  700 South Washington St.
  Suite 300
  Alexandria, VA 22314
  703-739-3900
  www.schoolnutrition.org

Team Nutrition
  U.S. Department of Agriculture, Food and Nutrition Service
  3101 Park Center Drive, Room 632
  Alexandria, VA 22302
  703-305-1624
  www.fns.usda.gov/tn

Web Sites

Sites for Kids:

Body and Mind
www.bam.gov

Dole 5-A-Day Site
www.dole5aday.com

Kidnetic
www.kidnetic.com

Kids Health
www.kidshealth.org/kid

Nutrition Cafe Game
www.exhibits.pacsci.org/nutrition

Science 4 Kids (from the Agricultural Research Service)
www.ars.usda.gov/is/kids/index.html

Smart-Mouth (a great interactive nutrition site)
www.smart-mouth.org

Verb: It's what you do (an activity based site for kids)
www.verbnow.com/

Nutrition Resources:

Action for Healthy Kids
   www.actionforhealthykids.org/

Communicating Food for Health Newsletter
   www.foodandhealth.com

Children's Nutrition Research Center — Baylor College of Medicine
   www.bcm.tmc.edu/cnrc

Dietary Guidelines for Americans 2005
   www.healthierus.gov/dietaryguidelines/

Eating Disorder Referral and Information Center
   www.edreferral.com

Iowa State Extension
   www.extension.iastate.edu/foodsafety

Nutrition Explorations
   www.nutritionexplorations.org

Nutrition for Kids (sponsored by 24 Carrot Press)
   www.nutritionforkids.com

Nutrition.gov
   www.nutrition.gov

University of Nebraska Cooperative Extension
   lancaster.unl.edu/food/

Nutrition/Health Sites for Teachers:

California Foundation for Agriculture in the Classroom
www.cfaitc.org

Healthteacher.com
www.healthteacher.com

Healthy Kids Challenge
www.healthykidschallenge.com

Healthy Start
www.Healthy-Start.com

Teachfree
teachfree.com

Bibliography

CHAPTER 1

Alaimo K, Olson CM, Frongillo Jr, EA. Food insufficiency and American school-aged children's cognitive, academic, and psychosocial development. *Pediatrics*. 2001;108:44–53.

American Academy of Pediatrics, Committee on Nutrition. Calcium requirements of of infants, children and adolescents. *Pediatrics*. 1999;104:1152–1157.

Andersen RE, Crespo CJ, Bartlett SJ, Cheskin LJ, Pratt M. Relationship of physical activity and television watching with body weight and level of fatness among children: results from the Third National Health and Nutrition Examination Survey. *JAMA*. 1998;279:938–42.

Basiotis PP, Carlson A, Gerrior SA., Juan WY, Lino M. The Healthy Eating Index: 1999–2000. U.S. Department of Agriculture, Center for Nutrition Policy and Promotion. 2002;CNPP-12. *www.usda.gov/cnpp/Pubs/HEI/HEI99–00report.pdf*, Accessed 2/03.

Basiotis PP, Lino M, Anand RS. Eating Breakfast Greatly Improves Schoolchildren's Diet Quality. Nutrition Insights; U.S. Department of Agriculture, Center for Nutrition Policy and Promotion. 1999; Insight 15. *www.usda.gov/cnpp/insights.html*, Accessed 2/03.

Bowman, SA. Beverage choices of young females: changes and impact on nutrient intakes. *J Am Diet Assoc*. 2002;102:1234–1239.

Carlson A, Lino M, Gerrior S, Basiotis PP. Report Card on the Diet Quality of Children Ages 2 to 9. Nutrition Insights; U.S. Department of Agriculture, Center for Nutrition Policy and Promotion. 2001; Insight 25. *www.usda.gov/cnpp/insights.html*, Accessed 2/03.

CSFII 1994-96, 1998 Data Set. Table set 17 (Food and Nutrient Intakes by Children 1994-96, 1998). *www.barc.usda.gov/bhnrc/foodsurvey*, Accessed 01/03.

Division of Adult and Community Health, National Center for Chronic Disease Prevention and Health Promotion, Centers for Disease Control and Prevention. Behavioral Risk Factor Surveillance System Online Prevalence Data, 1995-2000. *apps.nccd.cdc.gov/5ADaySurveillance*, Accessed 2/03.

Fisher JO, Mitchell DC, Smiciklas-Wright H, Birch LL. Parental influences on young girls' fruit and vegetable, micronutrient, and fat intakes. *J Am Diet Assoc.* 2002;102:58-64.

Gillman MW, Rifas-Shiman SL, Frazier AL, Rockett HRH, Camargo, Jr CA, Field AE, Berkey CS, Colditz GA. Family Dinner and Diet Quality Among Older Children and Adolescents. *Arch Fam Med.* 2000;9:235-240.

Hedley AA, Ogden CL, Johnson CL, Carroll MD, Curtin LR, Flegal KM. Prevalence of overweight and obesity among U.S. children, adolescents, and adults, 1999-2002. *JAMA* 2004;291(23):2847-2850.

Harnack L, Stang J, Story M. Soft drink consumption among US children and adolescents: nutritional consequences. *J Am Diet Assoc.* 1999;99:436-41.

Household Food Security in the United States, 2001, Food Assistance and Nutrition Research Report #29, Economic Research Service, U.S. Department of Agriculture 2002; *www.ers.usda.gov/publications/fanrr29*, Accessed 2/03.

Jahns L, Siega-Riz AM, Popkin BM. The increasing prevalence of snacking among US children from 1977 to 1996. *Journal of Pediatrics.* 2001;138:493-8.

Lino M, Gerrior SA, Basiotis PP, Anand, RS. Report card on the diet quality of children. Nutrition Insights; U.S. Department of Agriculture, Center for Nutrition Policy and Promotion. 1998; Insight 9. *www.usda.gov/cnpp/insights.html*, Accessed 2/03.

Ludwig D, Peterson K, Gortmaker S. Relationship between consumption of sugar-sweetened drinks and childhood obesity: A prospective, observational analysis. *Lancet*. 2001;358:505-508.

Murphy JM, Wehler CA, Pagano ME, Little M, Kleinman RE, Jellinek MS. Relationship between hunger and psychosocial functioning in low-income American children. *J Am. Acad. Child Adolesc Psychiatry*. 1998;37:163-170.

National Center for Chronic Disease Prevention and Health Promotion, Centers for Disease Control and Prevention. Physical Activity and Health: A Report of the Surgeon General, Adolescents and Young Adults. 1999.

National Center for Health Statistics. Prevalence of Overweight Among Children and Adolescents: United States, 1999. 2001; *www.cdc.gov/nchs/products/pubs/pubd/hestats/overwght99.htm*. Accessed 2/03.

Nielsen SJ, Popkin BM. Patterns and trends in food portion sizes, 1977-1998. *JAMA*. 2003;289:450-453.

Ogden CL, Flegal KM, Carroll MD, Johnson CL. Prevalence and trends in overweight among US children and adolescents, 1999-2000. *JAMA*. 2002;288:1728-32.

Rampersaud GC, Bailey LB, Kauwell GP. National survey beverage consumption data for children and adolescents indicate the need to encourage a shift toward more nutritive beverages. *J Am Diet Assoc*. 2003;103:97-100.

Rolls BJ. Engell D. Birch LL. Serving portion size influences 5-year-old but not 3-year-old children's food intakes. *J Am Diet Assoc.* 2000;100:232-234.

Sinha R, Fisch G, Teague B, Tamborlane WV, Banyas B, Allen K, Savoye M, Rieger V, Taksali S, Barbetta G, Sherwin RS, Caprio S. Prevalence of impaired glucose tolerance among children and adolescents with marked obesity. *N Engl J Med.* 2002;346:802-10.

Smiciklas-Wright H, Mitchell DC, Mickle SJ, Goldman JD, Cook A. Foods commonly eaten in the United States, 1989-1991 and 1994-1996: Are portion sizes changing? *J Am Diet Assoc.* 2003;103:41-47.

U.S. Department of Agriculture, Agricultural Research Service. Pyramid Servings Intakes by U.S. Children and Adults, 1994-1996, 1998. 2000;ARS Community Nutrition Research Group Web site. *www.barc.usda.gov/bhnrc/cnrg,* Accessed 2/03.

U.S. Department of Agriculture, Human Nutrition Information Service. The Interactive Healthy Eating Index. *www.usda.gov/cnpp,* Accessed 6/03.

U.S. Department of Education, National Center for Education Statistics. Nutrition Education in Public Elementary School Classrooms. 2000;NCES 2000-040. *nces.ed.gov/pubs2000/2000040.pdf,* Accessed 2/03.

Young LR, Nestle M. The contribution of expanding portion sizes to the U.S. obesity epidemic. *Am J Pub Hlth.* 2002;92:246-249.

Chapter 2

Abramovitz BA, Birch LL. Five-year-old girls' ideas about dieting are predicted by their mothers' dieting. *J Am Diet Assoc.* 2000;100:1157-1163.

Basiotis PP, Lino M, Anand RS. Eating Breakfast Greatly Improves
 Schoolchildren's Diet Quality. Nutrition Insights; U.S. Department of
 Agriculture, Center for Nutrition Policy and Promotion. 1999; Insight 15.
 www.usda.gov/cnpp/insights.html, Accessed 2/03.

Borzekowski DL, Robinson TN. The 30-second effect: An experiment
 revealing the impact of television commercials on food preferences of
 preschoolers. *J Am Diet Assoc.* 2001;101:42-46.

Byrd-Bredbenner C, Murray J. A longitudinal analysis of weight and shape
 ideals as defined by Miss America pageant winners. *J Am Diet Assoc.*
 2002;S102:A-73.

Consumers Union Education Services. Captive Kids:
 A Report on Commercial Pressures on Kids at School. 1995.
 www.consumersunion.org/other/captivekids/index.htm,
 Accessed 3/03.

Consumers Union Education Services. Selling America's Kids: Commercial
 Pressures on Kids of the 90's. 1990.

Coon KA, Goldberg J, Rogers BL, Tucker KL. Relationships
 Between Use of Television During Meals and Children's Food
 Consumption Patterns. *Pediatrics* 2001;107:E7.
 www.pediatrics.org/cgi/content/abstract/107/1/e7,
 Accessed 2/03.

Coon KA, Tucker KL. Television and children's consumption patterns.
 A review of the literature. *Minerva Pediatr* 2002;4:423-36.

Davis J, Oswalt R. Societal influences on a thinner body size in children.
 Percept Mot Skills. 1992;74:697-698.

Energizing the Classroom: A Summary of the Three Year Study of the Universal School Breakfast Pilot Program in Minnesota Elementary Schools. Available on the web at *www.nal.usda.gov/fnic/schoolmeals/States/energize.pdf*, Accessed 3/03.

Evers, C. Empower children to develop healthful eating habits. *J Am Diet Assoc.* 1997;S2:S116.

Field AE, Camargo CA Jr, Taylor CB, Berkey CS, Roberts SB, Colditz GA. Peer, parent, and media influences on the development of weight concerns and frequent dieting among preadolescent and adolescent girls and boys. *Pediatrics.* 2001;107:54-60.

Field AE, Cheung L, Wolf AM, Herzog DB, Gortmaker SL, Colditz GA. Exposure to the mass media and weight concerns among girls. *Pediatrics.* 1999;103:E36.

Fisher JO, Birch LL. Restricting access to palatable foods affects children's behavioral response, food selection, and intake. *Am J Clin Nutr* 1999;69:1264-72.

Fisher JO, Mitchell DC, Smiciklas-Wright H, Birch LL. Parental influences on young girls' fruit and vegetable, micronutrient, and fat intakes. *J Am Diet Assoc.* 2002;102:58-64.

Gallo, Anthony. "Food Advertising in the United States," in E. Frazao (ed.) America's Eating Habits: Changes and Consequences. USDA Economic Research Service, 1999.

Gustafson-Larson AM, Terry RD. Weight-related behaviors and concerns of fourth-grade children. *J Am Diet Assoc.* 1992;92:818-822.

Hogan M. Media Education Offers Help on Children's Body Image Problems. American Academy of Pediatrics, AAP News. May 1999;Online at *www.aap.org/advocacy/hogan599.htm*, Accessed 3/03.

Kotz K, Story M. Food advertisements during children's Saturday morning television programming: Are they consistent with dietary recommendations? *J Am Diet Assoc.* 1994;94:1296–1300.

Mackenzie M. Is the family meal disappearing? *J Gastronomy.* 1993;7:35–45.

McCabe MP, Ricciardelli LA. Parent, peer, and media influences on body image and strategies to both increase and decrease body size among adolescent boys and girls. *Adolescence.* 2001;36:225–40.

McLellan F. Marketing and advertising: harmful to children's health. *Lancet.* 2002;360:1001.

Mellin LM, Irwin CE, Scully S. Prevalence of disordered eating in girls: A survey of middle-class children. *J Am Diet Assoc.* 1992;92:851–853.

Neumark-Sztainer D, Sherwood NE, Coller T, Hannan PJ. Primary prevention of disordered eating among preadolescent girls: feasibility and short-term effect of a community-based intervention. *J Am Diet Assoc.* 2000;100:1466–73.

Pierce JW, Wardle J. Self-esteem, parental appraisal and body size in children. *J Child Psychol Psychiatry.* 1993;34:1125–1136.

Robinson TN. Reducing children's television viewing to prevent obesity: A randomized controlled trial. *JAMA.* 1999;282:1561–1567.

U.S. Department of Health and Human Services and U.S. Department of Agriculture. *Dietary Guidelines for Americans,* 2005. 6th edition, Washington, DC: U.S. Government Printing Office, January 2005.

U.S. Department of Agriculture, Center for Nutrition Policy and Promotion. MyPyramid.gov. April 2005.

CHAPTER 3

Hearn MD, Baranowski T, Baranowski J, Doyle C, Smith M, Lin LS, Resnicow K. Environmental influences on dietary behavior among children: availability and accessibility of fruits and vegetables enable consumption. *J Health Ed.* 1998;29:26-32.

Kelder SH, Perry CL, Klepp KI, Lytle L. Longitudinal tracking of adolescent smoking, physical activity, and food choice behaviors. *Am J Public Health.* 1994;84:1121-1126.

Liquori T, Koch PD, Contento IR, Castle J. The Cookshop Program: outcome evaluation of a nutrition education program linking lunchroom food experiences with classroom cooking experiences. *J Nutr Ed.* 1998;30:302-13.

Lytle, LA. Nutrition education for school-aged children: a review of research. USDA, Food and Consumer Service, Office of Analysis and Evaluation, September 1994.

Lytle, LA. Nutrition Education for School-Aged Children. *J Nutr Ed,* 1995;27:298-311.

Murphy AS, Youatt JP, Hoerr SL, Sawyer CA, Andrews SL. Nutrition education needs and learning preferences of Michigan students in grades 5, 8 and 11. *J Sch Health.* 1994:64:273-278.

Nader PR, Stone EJ, Lytle LA, Perry CL, Osganian SK, Kelder S, Webber LS, Elder JP, Montgomery D, Feldman HA, Wu M, Johnson C, Parcel GS, Luepker RV. Three-year maintenance of improved diet and physical activity: the CATCH cohort. Child and Adolescent Trial for Cardiovascular Health. *Arch Pediatr Adolesc Med.* 1999;53:695-704.

Perez-Escamilla R, Haldeman L, Gray S. Assessment of nutrition education needs in an urban school district in Connecticut: establishing priorities through research. *J Am Diet Assoc.* 2002 Apr;102:559-62.

Perry CL, Bishop DB, Taylor G, Murray DM, Mays RW, Dudovitz BS, Smyth M, Story M. Changing fruit and vegetable consumption among children: the 5-a-Day Power Plus Program in St. Paul, Minnesota. *Am J Publ Health.* 1998;88:603-9.

Position of the American Dietetic Association, Society for Nutrition Education, and American School Food Service Association – Nutrition services: an essential component of comprehensive school health programs. *J Am Diet Assoc.* 2003;103:505-514.

Simons-Morton BG, Parcel GS, Baranowski T, Forthofer R, O'Hara NM. Promoting physical activity and a healthful diet among children: results of a school-based intervention study. *Am J Public Health.* 1991;81:986-991.

Thomas LF, Long EM, Zaske JM. Nutrition education sources and priorities of elementary school teachers. *J Am Diet Assoc.* 1994;94:318-320.

U.S. Department of Agriculture, Food and Consumer Service, Office of Analysis and Evaluation. Charting the Course for Evaluation: How do we measure the success of nutrition education and promotion in food assistance programs? Summary of Proceedings. February, 1997.

U.S. Department of Education, National Center for Education Statistics. Nutrition Education in Public Elementary School Classrooms. 2000;NCES 2000-040. *nces.ed.gov/pubs2000/2000040.pdf,* Accessed 2/03.

CHAPTER 4

Carlson A, Mancino L, Lino M. Grain consumption by Americans. Nutrition Insights; U.S. Department of Agriculture, Center for Nutrition Policy and Promotion. 2005; Insight 32. www.usda.gov/cnpp/insights.html, Accessed 2/06.

Craig WJ. Phytochemicals: guardians of our health. *J Am Diet Assoc.* 1997;S2:S199–204.

Functional Foods for Health (FFH), a joint program of the University of Illinois at Chicago and the University of Illinois at Urbana–Champaign, *www.ag.uiuc.edu/~ffh*, Accessed 6/03.

King A, Young G. Characteristics and occurrence of phenolic phytochemicals. *J Am Diet Assoc.* 1999;99:213–8.

Position of the American Dietetic Association: functional foods. *J Am Diet Assoc.* 1999;99:1278–85.

Slavin J, Jacobs D, Marquart L, Wiemer K. The Role of Whole Grains in Disease Prevention *J Am Diet Assoc.* 2001;101:780–785. '

Health and Human Services and U.S. Department of Agriculture. *Dietary Guidelines for Americans*, 2005. 6th edition, Washington, DC: U.S. Government Printing Office, January 2005.

U.S. Department of Agriculture, Center for Nutrition Policy and Promotion. MyPyramid.gov. April 2005.

CHAPTER 5

U.S. Department of Agriculture, Center for Nutrition Policy and Promotion. MyPyramid.gov. April 2005.

Children's books:

Berenstain S, Berenstain J. *The Berenstain Bears and Too Much Junk Food.* Random House, 1985.

Brown M. *Stone Soup.* Scott Foresman, 1997.

Carle E. *The Very Hungry Caterpillar.* Scholastic, 1994.

Child L. *I Will Never Not Ever Eat a Tomato.* Candlewick Press, 2000.

Conford E. *What's Cooking, Jenny Archer?* Little, Brown, and Co., 1991.

Cook DF. *The Kids' Multicultural Cookbook: Food & Fun Around the World.* Williamson Publishing, 1995.

Cosgrove S. *Gobble and Gulp.* Random House, 1985.

D'Amico J, Drummond KE. *The Healthy Body Cookbook: Over 50 Fun Activities and Delicious Recipes for Kids,* John Wiley, 1999.

D'Amico J, Drummond KE. *The Science Chef Travels Around the World: Fun Food Experiments and Recipes for Kids.* John Wiley, 1996.

DeClements B. *Nothing's Fair in Fifth Grade.* Puffin, 1990.

deGroat D. *Annie Pitts, Artichoke.* SeaStar Books, 2001.

Diakité BW. *The Hatseller and the Monkeys.* Scholastic, 1999.

Dr. Seuss. *Green Eggs and Ham.* Random House, 1960.

Ehlert L. *Eating the Alphabet: Fruits & Vegetables From A to Z.* Voyager Books, 1993.

French V. *Oliver's Fruit Salad.* Orchard Books, 1998.

French V. *Oliver's Milkshake.* Orchard Books, 2001.

French V. *Oliver's Vegetables*. Orchard Books, 1995.

Gretz S. *Rabbit Food*. Candlewick Press, 1999.

Haduch B, Stromoski R. *Food Rules! The Stuff You Munch, Its Crunch, Its Punch, and Why You Sometimes Lose Your Lunch*. Puffin Books, 2001.

Hoban R. *Bread and Jam for Frances*. HarperTrophy, 1993.

Janovitz M. *Good Morning, Little Fox*. North-South Books, 2001.

Johmann CA, Rieth E. *Gobble Up Science*. Learning Works, 1996.

McCloskey R. *Blueberries for Sal*. Puffin, 1976.

McMillan B. *Eating Fractions*. Scholastic Inc., 1991.

Mogard S, McDonnell G. *Gobble Up Math*. Learning Works, 1994.

Ottolenghi C, Holladay R. *The Little Red Hen*. McGraw-Hill Childrens Publishing, 2001.

Park B. *Junie B. Jones, First Grader: Boss of Lunch*. Random House, 2002.

Passen L. *Fat, Fat Rose Marie*. Henry Holt, 1991.

Rayner, M. *Mrs. Pig's Bulk Buy*. Atheneum, 1990.

Rockwell L. *Good Enough to Eat: A Kid's Guide to Food and Nutrition*. HarperCollins, 1999.

Sharmat M. *Gregory the Terrible Eater*. Scholastic, 1989.

Sturges P. *The Little Red Hen (Makes a Pizza!)*. Dutton Children's Books, 1999.

Todd P. *Pig and the Shrink*. Delacorte Press, 1999.

Vancleave JP. *Janice Vancleave's Food and Nutrition for Every Kid: Easy Activities That Make Learning Science Fun*. John Wiley, 1999.

CHAPTER 6

Department of Food Science and Human Nutrition, University of Illinois (Urbana-Champaign). Nutritional Analysis Tool (NAT). *www.nat.uiuc.edu/mainnat.html*, Accessed 7/03.

U.S. Department of Agriculture, Center for Nutrition Policy and Promotion. MyPyramid Tracker. *www.mypyramidtracker.gov*, Accessed 2/06.

U.S. Department of Health and Human Services, U.S. Food and Drug Administration, and Center for Food Safety and Applied Nutrition. Food labeling and nutrition. *vm.cfsan.fda.gov/label.html*, Accessed 7/03.

U.S. Department of Health and Human Services, U.S. Food and Drug Administration. FDA acts to provide better information to consumers on trans fats. *www.fda.gov/oc/initiatives/transfat*, Accessed 7/03.

CHAPTER 7

Getlinger MJ, Laughlin CVT, Bell E, Akre C, Arjmandi BH. Food waste is reduced when elementary-school children have recess before lunch. *J Am Diet Assoc.* 1996:96:906-908.

Morris J, Zidenberg-Cherr S. Garden-enhanced nutrition curriculum improves fourth-grade schoolchildren's knowledge of nutrition and preferences for some vegetables. *J Am Diet Assoc.* 2002;102:24-30.

Morris JL, Koumjian K, Briggs M, Zidenburg-Cherr S. Nutrition to grow on: A garden-enhanced nutrition education curriculum for upper-elementary school children. *J Nutr Educ Behav.* 2002;34:175-176.

National Gardening Association. www.kidsgardening.com, Accessed 7/03.

Patten E, Lyons K. Healthy foods from healthy soils. Tilbury House Publishers, 2003.

Smith DV, Margolskee, RF. Making sense of taste. *Scientific American*. March, 2001.

U.S. Department of Agriculture, Agricultural Research Service. 2002. USDA National Nutrient Database for Standard Reference, Release 15. Nutrient Data Laboratory Home Page, *www.nal.usda.gov/fnic/foodcomp*, Accessed 7/03.

Webb FS, Whitney EN. *Nutrition Concepts and Controversies*. Wadsworth Publishing, 2002.

Children's Books:

Epstein S, Epstein B. *Dr. Beaumont and the Man with the Hole In His Stomach*. Coward, McCann and Geoghegan, 1978.

Showers P. *What Happens to a Hamburger*. HarperCollins Juvenile Books, 2001.

Swanson D. Burp! *The Most Interesting Book You'll Ever Read About Eating*. Kids Can Press, 2001.

CHAPTER 8

Birch LL. Children's eating: are manners enough? *J Gastronomy*. 1993;7:19–25.

Cox B, Jacobs M, Weatherford J. *Spirit of the Earth: Cooking from Latin America*. Stewart, Tabori, & Chang, 2001.

Derrickson JP, Widodo MME, Jarosz LA. Providers of food to homeless and hungry people need more dairy, fruit, vegetable, and lean-meat items. J Am Diet Assoc. 1994;94:445–446.

Frank LE. *Foods of the Southwest Indian Nations: Traditional & Contemporary Native American Recipes*. Ten Speed Press, 2002.

Fussell B. *The Story of Corn*. Alfred A Knoff, 1992.

Lavine SA. *Indian Corn and Other Gifts*. Dodd, Mead and Co., 1974.

Mackenzie M. Is the family meal disappearing? *J Gastronomy*. 1993;7:35–45.

Mintz SW. Feeding, eating, and grazing: some speculations on modern food habits. *J Gastronomy*. 1993;7:46–57.

Stefkovich C. The value of diversity. *School Food Serv Nutr*. 1994;October:61–63.

U.S. Department of Agriculture, Economic Research Service. Household Food Security in the United States, 2001. Food Assistance and Nutrition Research Report #29. November 2002, *www.ers.usda.gov/publications/fanrr29*, Accessed 2/03.

Children's Books:

Albyn CL, Webb LS. *The Multicultural Cookbook for Students*. Oryx Press, 1993.

Aliki. *Corn is Maize: The Gift of the Indians*. HarperTrophy, 1986.

Badt KL. *Good Morning, Let's Eat!* Children's Press, 1994.

Bial R. *Corn Belt Harvest*. Houghton Mifflin, 1991.

Cook DF. *The Kids' Multicultural Cookbook: Food & Fun Around the World*. Williamson Publishing, 2003.

Cutler J. *Family Dinner*. Sunburst, 1995.

Dooley N. *Everybody Bakes Bread*. Carolrhoda Books, 1996.

Dooley N. *Everybody Brings Noodles*. Carolrhoda Books, 2002.

Dooley N. *Everybody Cooks Rice*. Scott Foresman,1992

Dooley N. *Everybody Serves Soup*. Carolrhoda Books, 2000.

Friedman IR. *How My Parents Learned to Eat*. Houghton Mifflin, 1987.

Gershator D, Gershator P. *Bread is for Eating*. Henry Holt & Co., Inc., 1995.

Kandoian E. *Is Anybody Up?* Putnam Pub Group, 1989.

Kellogg C. *Corn: What it is, What it Does*. Greenwillow, 1989.

Lauber P, Manders J. *What You Never Knew About Fingers, Forks and Chopsticks*. Aladdin Library, 2002.

Lin G. *The Ugly Vegetables*. Charlesbridge Publishing, 1999.

Shelby A. *Potluck*. Orchard Books, 1991.

CHAPTER 9

Coon KA, Tucker KL. Television and children's consumption patterns. A review of the literature. *Minerva Pediatr* 2002;54:423-36.

Gallo A. Food advertising in the United States. In: Frazao E, ed. America's Eating Habits: Changes and Consequences. USDA Economic Research Service, 1999.

Gay K. *Caution! This May Be An Advertisement (A Teen Guide to Advertising)*. Franklin Watts, 1992.

McLellan F. Marketing and advertising: harmful to children's health. *Lancet*. 2002;360:1001.

Perry CL, Zauner M, Oakes JM, Taylor G, Bishop DB. Evaluation of a theater production about eating behavior of children. *J Sch Health* 2002;72:256-61.

Children's Books:

deGroat D. *Annie Pitts, Artichoke*. SeaStar Books, 2001.

Wake S. *Advertising: Media Story*. Garrett Educational Corporation, 1990

CHAPTER 11

Andersen RE, Crespo CJ, Bartlett SJ, Cheskin LJ, Pratt M. Relationship of physical activity and television watching with body weight and level of fatness among children: results from the Third National Health and Nutrition Examination Survey. *JAMA*. 1998;279:938-42.

Fisher B, Hopper C, Munoz K. Fitting in fitness: an integrated approach to health, nutrition, and exercise. *Learning91*. 1991;July/August:25-54.

Frequency and Intensity of Activity of Third-Grade Children in Physical Education,The National Institute of Child Health and Human Development Study of Early Child Care and Youth Development Network, *Arch Pediatr Adolesc Med*. 2003;157:185-190. *www.nichd.nih.gov/new/releases/exercise.cfm*, Accessed 3/03.

Johnson C. Taking the classroom beyond four walls. *Newsletter of Oregon Association of the Advancement of Health Education (OAAHE)*. Spring, 1989.

Kimm SY, Glynn NW, Kriska AM, Barton BA, Kronsberg SS, Daniels SR, Crawford PB, Sabry ZI, Liu K. Decline in physical activity in black girls and white girls during adolescence. *N Engl J Med*. 2002;347:709-715. *www.nih.gov/news/pr/sep2002/nhlbi-04.htm*, Accessed 3/03.

National Cholesterol Education Program Coordinating Committee. Report of the Expert Panel on Blood Cholesterol in Children and Adolescents. Bethesda, Md: National Heart, Lung and Blood Institute. NIH Publication no. 91-2732. 1991.

PDAY Research Group. Natural history of aortic and coronary atherosclerotic lesions in youth: Findings from the PDAY study. *Arterioscler Thromb.* 1993;13:1291–1298.

Physical Activity and Health: A Report of the Surgeon General, Adolescents and Young Adults, National Center for Chronic Disease Prevention and Health Promotion, Centers for Disease Control and Prevention, 1999.

State study proves physically fit kids perform better academically. California Department of Education News Release, December 10, 2002, *www.cde.ca.gov/nr/ne/yr02/yr02rel37.asp*, Accessed 2/06.

Williams MH. Exercise effects on children's health. Sports Science Exchange. The Gatorade Sports Science Institute, March 1993.

CHAPTER 12

American Dietetic Association. Local support for nutrition integrity in schools - position of ADA. *J Am Diet Assoc.* 2000;100:108–111.

American School Food Service Association. Keys of Excellence: Standards of Practice for Nutrition Integrity. Alexandra, VA: American School Food Service Association; 1995:29–36.

Coddington RM. A "NAC" for excitement. *School Food Serv J.* 1995;January:45–48.

Evers C. A nutrition education report card. *School Foodservice & Nutrition.* 2000;June/July:22–30.

Evers C. More nutrition, less waste. *School Foodservice & Nutrition.* 1995;November:76.

Fox MK, Crepinek MK, Connor P, Battaglia M. School Nutrition Dietary Assessment Study-II: Summary of Findings. US Dept of Agriculture Office of Analysis, Nutrition and Evaluation. Report No. CN-00-SNDAII; 2001.

Harding Lawson Associates. Offer Versus Serve and Food Choices in Elementary School Cafeterias: Waste Prevention Pilot Projects at North Plains Elementary School, Charles F. Tigard Elementary School, and Metzger Elementary School, Unpublished data, May 1994.

Kubik MY, Lytle LA, Story M. A practical, theory-based approach to establishing school nutrition advisory councils. *J Am Diet Assoc.* 2001;101:223-228.

Position of the American Dietetic Association, Society for Nutrition Education, and American School Food Service Association – Nutrition services: an essential component of comprehensive school health programs. *J Am Diet Assoc.* 2003;103:505-514.

U.S. Department of Agriculture Office of Food and Nutrition Services. Foods Sold in Competition with USDA School Meal Programs: A Report to Congress. Washington, DC: WSDA; January 2001.

U.S. Department of Health and Human Services. Healthy People 2010: Understanding and Improving Health. 2nd ed. Washington, DC: US Government Printing Office; November 2000.

Index

THE AUTHOR

Connie Evers, M.S., R.D. is a registered dietitian, consultant and author who specializes in the health of children and adolescents. She works as a nutrition education consultant to schools, universities, state agencies and USDA child nutrition programs, and is a frequent guest on radio and television programs throughout the U.S. She lives in Portland, Oregon with her husband, three children and "Lady" the dog.

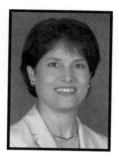

THE DESIGNER/ILLUSTRATOR

Carol Buckle has many years of creative nutrition education experience in both the public and private sector and has collaborated with Connie Evers on numerous books, projects and school curricula. She is the recipient of local and national awards for her work. She lives in Portland, Oregon and is a senior partner in the communication design firm Anderson Buckle Creative.

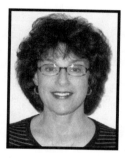

ORDER FORM

HOW TO TEACH NUTRITION TO KIDS ISBN 0964797011
_____copies at $19.95 per copy $_____

Shipping & Handling
$4.00 per book for 1st book; $1.00 for each additional book $_____

TOTAL ENCLOSED $_____

Name/Affiliation_____

Address _____

City _____ State_____ Zip_____

Telephone_____ Fax_____

Email _____

MasterCard/Visa: _____ Exp.Date:_____

Authorized Signature _____

Send payment to: 24 CARROT PRESS, P.O. Box 23546, Portland, OR 97281-3546;
Phone/Fax: 503-524-9318;

Order online at _http://www.nutritionforkids.com_. **Quantity Discounts Available – Call for rates.**

HOW TO TEACH NUTRITION TO KIDS ISBN 0964797011
_____copies at $19.95 per copy $_____

Shipping & Handling
$4.00 per book for 1st book; $1.00 for each additional book $_____

TOTAL ENCLOSED $_____

Name/Affiliation_____

Address _____

City _____ State_____ Zip_____

Telephone_____ Fax_____

Email _____

MasterCard/Visa: _____ Exp.Date:_____

Authorized Signature _____

Send payment to: 24 CARROT PRESS, P.O. Box 23546, Portland, OR 97281-3546;
Phone/Fax: 503-524-9318;

Order online at _http://www.nutritionforkids.com_. **Quantity Discounts Available – Call for rates.**

ORDER FORM

HOW TO TEACH NUTRITION TO KIDS ISBN 0964797011
_____copies at $19.95 per copy $_____

Shipping & Handling
$4.00 per book for 1st book; $1.00 for each additional book $_____

TOTAL ENCLOSED $_____

Name/Affiliation_____

Address _____

City _____ State____ Zip_____

Telephone_____ Fax_____

Email _____

MasterCard/Visa: _____ Exp.Date:_____

Authorized Signature _____

Send payment to: 24 CARROT PRESS, P.O. Box 23546, Portland, OR 97281-3546;
Phone/Fax: 503-524-9318;

Order online at _http://www.nutritionforkids.com_. **Quantity Discounts Available – Call for rates.**

HOW TO TEACH NUTRITION TO KIDS ISBN 0964797011
_____copies at $19.95 per copy $_____

Shipping & Handling
$4.00 per book for 1st book; $1.00 for each additional book $_____

TOTAL ENCLOSED $_____

Name/Affiliation_____

Address _____

City _____ State____ Zip_____

Telephone_____ Fax_____

Email _____

MasterCard/Visa: _____ Exp.Date:_____

Authorized Signature _____

Send payment to: 24 CARROT PRESS, P.O. Box 23546, Portland, OR 97281-3546;
Phone/Fax: 503-524-9318;

Order online at _http://www.nutritionforkids.com_. **Quantity Discounts Available – Call for rates.**